Acumoxa Therapy II

Acumoxa Therapy

A Reference and Study Guide

—II—

The Treatment of Disease

Paul Zmiewski and Richard Feit

Paradigm Publications   Brookline, Massachusetts

1990

Library of Congress Cataloging in Publication Data

Zmiewski, Paul
Acumoxa therapy.

Bibliography: p. 185-186
        Includes index.
        Contents: --v. 2. Treatment of disease.
        ISBN 0-912111-27-5 : $17.95
        1. Moxa. I. Feit, Richard. II. Title.
        RM306.Z55 1990   615.8'92   89-2989
ISBN 0-912111-22-4
ISBN 0-912111-27-5 (v. 2.)

Paradigm Publications

Publisher: Robert Felt
Editor: Richard Feit

Typesetting Software
by
Textware International, Cambridge, Massachusetts

Contents

"The marvel of the needle
lies in its subtlety."

— *Nan Jing 74*

Preface

This second volume of the *Acumoxa Therapy* review series takes the reader from the basic theories, systems, and structures of Chinese medicine presented in volume I to the application of those theories in the treatment of disease. As with the first volume of the series, this current volume is intended to accompany formal instruction, and to provide a source for ongoing review after formal instruction has been completed.

The treatment of disease is approached here from both traditional Chinese patterns and from Western disease categories. This dual approach is intended to coincide with the structure of most courses in acupuncture pathology, and reflects common clinical practice.

Part I of the text restates the traditional patterns of disharmony discussed in volume I, and adds the traditional methods of treatment and the representative points. That these point formulae are *representative* cannot be overemphasized. They are presented not so much as complete treatments (though they can be used as such), but as the foundation upon which individual approaches to therapy can be developed.

Approximately one hundred common disorders are presented according to Western disease categories in **Part II**. Guiding symptomatology, traditional Chinese medical differentiation, and appropriate points and treatments are also included. The locations of the points used are presented in the appendix.

The same table format used in volume I is used in volume II, facilitating study and cross-reference between both texts.

Please note that in all tables, the sign † indicates moxibustion.

Introduction

From Theory to Practice: Systematic Examination and Diagnosis

Diagnosis is the first, and often most bewildering, of the many hurdles that students must overcome in transposing theoretical understanding to practical application. In traditional Chinese medicine, becoming a skilled and accurate diagnostician makes life-long students of us all. Diagnosis itself is the distillate of the entire medical system, combining perceptual skills and physical and spiritual sensitivity with an understanding of suffering and the progression of illness.

While there is no substitute for clinical experience in this process, certain general principles guide the practitioner toward diagnostic proficiency. These guidelines are fundamental, and may be applied regardless of the particular style of acupuncture or Chinese medicine you choose to practice.

Recording, Organization, and Evaluation

A thorough and systematic examination is the key to an accurate diagnosis.

•*Keep an open mind* when gathering data. Though it is certainly important to take notice of first impressions, avoid being unduly biased by them. When you first encounter your patient, all you should be concerned with is obtaining information; arriving at a diagnosis comes much later. Be as thorough as possible, leaving no stone unturned. Since traditional Chinese diagnosis depends almost entirely upon observational data, there can be no substitute for, or short cut to, clarity of perception. This skill will ultimately determine the quality of the data used to arrive at a diagnosis.

•*Record all data* meticulously and impartially.

•*Organize your data* according to the eight parameters and/or the five phases.

When organizing data according to the eight parameters, first determine whether the disorder is generally yin or yang in character. At this point, yin and yang refer to the *general nature* of the illness—whether it is acute or chronic, hot or cold, spastic or flaccid, etc. Then classify signs and symptoms according to the remaining six parameters. This will determine the *general location* (surface vs. interior), the *symptomatic appearance* (hot vs. cold), and the *physioenergetic nature* (repletion vs. depletion) of the disorder. Now return to the principles of yin and yang to determine the *physiologic aspect* (qi vs. blood, *zang* vs. *fu*) affected.

Next, determine more precisely the *depth* and *severity* of the problem. If it is a surface problem, confirm which channels are affected, and their channel type. If it is an interior problem, determine whether it is at the level of organic interaction, triple burner metabolism, or a more general derangement of qi or blood. If the problem is due to an exogenous pathogen, determine the *level* of the body affected according to the six stages, the four aspects, or the three burning spaces.

When organizing data according to the the five phases, determine from the radial pulses which phase is most replete, and which phase is most deplete. Decide whether the imbalance may be attributed to an individual *zang* or *fu* organ, or whether combined *zang-fu* pairs are affected. Then verify your pulse diagnosis with observable evidence (complexion, emotion, tone of voice, etc.). If the pulse pattern does not coincide with observable evidence according to established principles, reconsider whether the disorder does in fact conform to a five-phase pattern.

•*Evaluate* all data in light of the patient's signs and symptoms. Determine what is primary and what is secondary. For example, if both *zang* and *fu* organs are affected, or both surface and interior, decide what is the root and what are the branches. If possible, determine the cause of the problem. If it is external in origin, determine the pathogenic factor(s) involved. If it is internal in origin, determine whether the cause is emotional, dietary, hereditary, or a residue from a previous external disruption. Furthermore, determine whether the cause still exists in the present reality of your patient's life. If it no longer exists, treat the situation as you see it. If it still exists, it will have to be taken into consideration when determining a treatment strategy.

Reaching a Working Diagnosis and Inferring a Treatment Principle

At this point, you can establish a *working diagnosis* and infer a *treatment principle*. A diagnosis should always include the *condition, location,* and *possible cause.*

A condition may be seen as a combination of the eight parameters, such as a replete, hot, interior condition, or a deplete, cold, surface condition, etc. The *disease location* refers to the physioenergetic level of the body affected: whether it is at the general level of yin or yang (i.e., blood or qi); whether it is in the upper, middle, or lower burner; whether it is affecting certain *zang* or *fu* organs; or whether it is at the level of the primary channels, connecting channels, or muscle channels. The cause may be inferred from the patient's history and the nature of the illness. Accurately determining the physioenergetic level of disease is often important for determining the correct therapeutic technique and preventing recurrence of the problem.

Never treat without first making a diagnosis. Avoid haphazardly treating symptom by symptom. Clearly identify, for yourself and for the patient, exactly what you believe to be the problem. If you have a clear idea of what you are treating, you will be able to form a coherent plan of action and follow it through. Once a working diagnosis is reached, a treatment principle can be easily inferred. A diagnosis of "depleted yang of the lower burner," for example, obviously implies the treatment principle of "supplementing yang of the lower burner."

Determining a Treatment Strategy

Once you have arrived at a diagnosis and inferred a treatment principle, determine a *treatment strategy*. A treatment strategy is based upon the application of your treatment principle to the specific physioenergetic level affected. Choose channels affecting the level primarily responsible for the problem; choose points along those channels that will affect functioning on that level according to the treatment principle indicated. Choose points that have a consistent, mutually supportive effect, according to channel circulation and functional interrelationships. Don't just haphazardly choose points that all seem to affect the "problem"; utilize the circulatory relationships of the arm and leg channel branches, *zang* and *fu* paired organs, five-phase interactions, irregular (extraordinary) vessel and primary channel correspondences, twenty-four hour cycle circulation, etc. Every treatment need not be "elegant," but at least it must be *sensible*.

Determine alternative treatment strategies. Human function may be affected from many directions; often, a less direct approach may be more appropriate, particularly in older people, or for more complex degenerative problems. Decide, also, what adjunctive therapies may effectively supplement treatment. Be sure, though, that such therapies do not interfere with the primary therapy; don't short-circuit your own treatment!

Advising the Patient

Explain your diagnosis clearly in terms your patient can understand. Try, also, to explain the rationale behind your strategy. The more your patient understands, the more he or she will cooperate with your treatment plan and lifestyle suggestions, and the greater will be your chances of success. Set up a treatment schedule that will conform both to *your* needs (in terms of maximum efficacy) and *the patient's* needs. No patient will cooperate with a treatment plan they perceive as too expensive or inconvenient. Remember that Chinese medical therapy continues beyond your acumoxa treatment: what your patient does outside your clinic will directly affect the outcome of your treatment.

Reassessment and Re-evaluation

Monitor your patient's progress with each successive treatment. Treatment is a *process* and diagnosis a *flexible assessment* of the patient's condition, which changes as the patient's condition improves, as his or her life situation changes, and as new factors emerge. Follow this process, modifying your treatments accordingly. Don't get stuck in your diagnosis. Don't be afraid to change your diagnosis or treatment strategy if your results are unsatisfactory. However, for long-term or difficult problems, remember that perseverence is vital. If, after a reasonable amount of time or number of treatments, you really seem to be going nowhere, don't give up: *reevaluate*. If necessary, consult with another practitioner for a different opinion or a fresh perspective. Within the realm of conditions treatable by acupuncture, there are few that will not yield to patience and persistence, on the part of both the patient and the practitioner.

Maintenance and Follow-up

As symptoms improve, extend the length of time between treatments, but even when the symptoms are relieved completely, have your patient return for periodic, constitutionally supportive treatments until you are satisfied that the problem will not recur. And even then, encourage your patient to come in for periodic "tune-ups," either monthly, bi-monthly, or at the change of seasons, according to the nature of the original problem and the strength of your patient's constitutional energy. Impress upon your patient that the absence of symptoms is only one treatment objective; restoration of total health is the ultimate goal.

Part I

Treatment Methods and Representative Points

	—Overview— Patterns of Illness	
Pattern Category	**Patterns**
Eight Parameter Patterns	Exterior and Interior Hot and Cold Repletion and Depletion Yang and Yin
Qi-Blood Patterns	Qi Depletion Patterns Qi Stagnation Patterns Qi Fall Patterns Qi Counterflow Patterns Blood Depletion Patterns Blood Stasis Patterns Blood Heat Patterns
Zang-fu Patterns	Heart (6), Lung (4), Spleen (3), Stomach/Spleen (4), Liver (10), Kidney (11), Stomach (3), Small Intestine (3), Large Intestine (2), Gallbladder (2), Bladder (2). *Numbers in parentheses indicate number of patterns presented*
Pathogen Patterns	Wind, Cold, Heat and Fire, Summerheat, Damp, Dryness, Digestate Accumulation, Phlegm
Exogenous Heat Patterns	*Six-Channel Patterns*: Taiyang, Shaoyang, Yangming, Taiyin, Shaoyin, Jueyin
	Four-Aspect Patterns: Defense (*wei*), Qi, Construction (*ying*), Blood
	Triple-Burner Patterns: Upper Burner (Lung and Pericardium) Middle Burner (Stomach and Spleen) Lower Burner (Liver and Kidney)
	Pericardiac Patterns: Inward Fall of Pathogens to the Pericardium Clouding of the Pericardium by Phlegm Turbidity Stomach Heat Sweltering the Pericardium

	—Overview— **Eight Common Treatment Methods**	
Method	**Summary**
Diaphoresis	Opening the striations to expel a pathogen from the body's surface
Clearage	Clearing and draining pathogenic heat
Ejection	Promoting emesis or phlegm ejection to expel pathogens or harmful substances in the stomach or lung
Precipitation	Stimulating fecal flow to expel repletion pathogens and remove accumulation and stagnation of substances
Harmonization	Adjusting disharmonies of qi and blood or among the organs
Warming	Supplementing yang qi to expel the cold pathogen
Supplementation	Supplying insufficiencies of yin and yang, blood and qi, or organic function
Dispersion	Draining replete pathogens in the qi or blood; dispersing accumulation or stagnation of qi or blood

1 Treatment of Eight-Parameter Patterns

—Overview— Patterns of Illness	
Eight-Parameter Patterns	Exterior, Interior, Hot, Cold, Repletion, Depletion, Yang, Yin

Exterior Patterns		
Pattern	**Method of Treatment**	**Representative Points**
Exterior Heat	Clear heat in the exterior	LI-4, LI-11, GV-14
Exterior Cold	Resolve cold in the exterior	LU-7, LI-4†, TB-5†
Exterior Repletion	Expel repletion pathogen	LI-4, TB-5, BL-12, GB-20, GV-16
Exterior Depletion	Harmonize construction and defense	LU-7, LI-4, ST-36

Interior Patterns

Pattern	Method of Treatment	Representative Points
Interior Heat	Clear heat from the interior	LI-11, GV-14, BL-40
Interior Cold	Warm the interior	CV-4†, CV-12†, ST-36†
Interior Repletion	Forcefully drain the interior pathogen	High Fever: M-UE-1 *to* -10 (bleed) Upper Burner: LU-7, BL-13, BL-15 Middle Burner: PC-6, BL-20, BL-21 Lower Burner: SP-6, ST-25, BL-25
Interior Depletion	Fortify and nourish blood	BL-17†, BL-19†, BL-43†, ST-36†, SP-6†

Heat Patterns *(with Depletion and Repletion)*

Pattern Type	Method of Treatment	Representative Points
Repletion Heat *(intense heat pathogen)*	Clear heat and drain fire	LI-11, GV-14, ST-44 Extreme Heat: KI-1 M-UE-1 *to* -10 (bleed)
Depletion Heat *(yin humor depletion)*	Nourish yin to clear heat	LU-7, KI-6, SP-6, CV-4

Cold Patterns *(with Depletion and Repletion)*

Pattern Type	Method of Treatment	Representative Points
Repletion Cold *(cold pathogen congestion)*	Warm and free repletion cold	CV-6†, CV-8† (on salt), CV-12†
Depletion Cold *(debilitation of yang qi)*	Warm yang and restore the correct	LI-4†, GV-14†, ST-36†

Repletion Patterns

Qi Repletion Patterns

Pattern	Method of Treatment	Representative Points
Lung Qi Repletion	Drain lungs and transform phlegm	PC-5, CV-22, CV-17, BL-13
Stomach Qi Repletion	Harmonize the stomach	CV-12, BL-21

Blood Repletion Patterns

Pattern	Method of Treatment	Representative Points
Blood Repletion	Quicken the blood and disperse stasis	LV-3, SP-8, SP-10, BL-18, BL-20
Internal Heat Repletion	Clear heat from the interior	Blood heat: SP-10, LI-11, BL-40 Channel heat: LI-4, LI-11, GV-14, ST-44
Internal Cold Repletion	Warm the center and dissipate cold	LI-4†, CV-12†, BL-20†, BL-21†, ST-36†

Depletion Patterns

Qi and Yang

Pattern	Method of Treatment	Representative Points
Qi Depletion	Reinforce qi	CV-4†, CV-6†, ST-36†
Yang Depletion	Warm yang	GV-4†, BL-12†, GV-14†

Blood and Yin

Pattern	Method of Treatment	Representative Points
Blood Depletion	Supplement the blood	BL-18, BL-20, ST-36
Yin Depletion	Enrich yin	KI-3, SP-6, CV-4, BL-23

Treating General Disturbances of Yin and Yang (Blood and Qi)	
Disturbance	**Treatment**
General repletion of yang	Supplement yin master points (PC-6, SP-4, LU-7, KI-6).
	Drain general points of yang (GV-14, GV-20, LI-4).
Yang repletion in the upper body	Supplement yin in upper body with yin master points (PC-6, LU-7).
	Supplement yang in lower body through group *luo* point (GB-39), and general point of yang (ST-36).
Yang repletion in the lower body	Supplement yin in lower body with yin master points (SP-4, KI-6).
	Supplement yang in upper body through group *luo* point (TB-8), and general point of yang (LI-4).
General repletion of yin	Supplement yang master points (TB-5, GB-41, SI-3, BL-62).
	Supplement general points of yang (GV-14, GV-20, LI-4, ST-30). Note that ST-30 may be supplemented, but not drained.
Yin repletion in the upper body	Supplement yang in upper body through yang master points (TB-5, SI-3).
	Supplement yin in lower body through group *luo* point (SP-6), and general point of yin (LV-3).
Yin repletion in the lower body	Supplement yang in lower body through yang master points (GB-41, BL-62).
	Supplement yin in upper body through group *luo* point (PC-5).

2 Treatment of Qi-Blood Patterns

Common Qi Depletion Patterns		
Pattern	**Treatment Method**	**Representative Points**
General Qi Depletion	Use master points of yang and general points of yang to supplement qi of the entire body	SI-3, TB-5, BL-62, GB-41, LI-4, ST-36, GV-1, GV-4
Lung Qi Depletion	Reinforce lung qi.	LU-9, BL-12, BL-13
	Fortify kidney qi	GV-4, BL-23
Heart Qi Depletion	Supplement heart qi; supplement the kidney or lung qi according to the symptoms	HT-9, HT-7, BL-15, BL-23, GV-4, LU-9, BL-13
Gastrosplenic Qi Depletion	Supplement gastrosplenic qi and regulate the colon	ST-36, SP-6, BL-20, BL-21, LI-4, CV-12, ST-25, ST-37

Common Blood Depletion Patterns		
Pattern	**Treatment Method**	**Representative Points**
General Blood Depletion	Use Master points of yin to supplement blood of the entire body, and supplement stomach and spleen to engender blood	LU-7, PC-6, KI-3, SP-4, ST-36, SP-6
Cardiosplenic Blood Depletion	Supplement the blood to nourish the heart	SP-6, BL-20, BL-17
Liver Blood Depletion	Nourish the liver and supplement the blood	LV-3, LV-8, LV-14, SP-6, SP-10, BL-17

3 Treatment of *Zang-Fu* Patterns

—Overview— Zang-Fu Patterns	
Organ	**Potential Disorders**
Heart	Heart Qi Depletion Heart Yang Depletion Heart Blood Depletion Heart Yin Depletion Upflaming of Heart Fire Cardiac *Bi*
Lung	Non-Diffusion of Lung Qi Impaired Depurative Downbearing of Lung Qi Lung Qi Depletion Lung Yin Depletion
Spleen	Spleen Qi Depletion Devitalization of Splenic Yang Center Qi Fall
Stomach/Spleen	Blood Management Failure Gastric Qi Depletion Cold Insufficiency of Stomach Yin
Liver	General Binding Depression of Liver Qi Invasion of the Stomach by Liver Qi Hepatosplenic Disharmony Plumstone Globus Struma Disorders of the Governing and Penetrating Vessels Upflaming of Liver Fire Ascendant Hyperactivity of Liver Yang Liver Wind Liver Blood Depletion

(Continued)

Zang-Fu Patterns
(Continued)

Organ	Potential Disorder
Kidney	Kidney Yin Depletion Cardiorenal Yin Depletion Hepatorenal Yin Depletion Pulmorenal Yin Depletion Kidney Yang Depletion Splenorenal Yang Depletion Qi-Absorption Failure Cardiorenal Yang Debilitation Yang Depletion Water Flood Insufficiency of Kidney Essence Insecurity of Kidney Qi
Stomach	Stomach Heat Stomach Yang Insufficiency Stomach Cold Stomach Qi Depletion Epigastric Food Stagnation
Small Intestine	Depletion Cold of the Small Intestine Repletion Heat of the Small Intestine Small Intestine Qi Pain
Large Intestine	Large Intestine Repletion Heat Large Intestine Damp Heat Large Intestine Fluid Depletion Intestinal Depletion Efflux Desertion Large Intestine Depletion Cold
Gallbladder	Gallbladder Repletion Gallbladder Depletion
Bladder	Bladder Damp Heat Bladder Depletion Cold

Heart Illness Patterns *(Depletion)*		
Pattern Type	**Method of Treatment**	**Representative Points**
Heart Qi Depletion	Supplement heart qi	HT-9, BL-15
	Nourish the heart and quiet the spirit	HT-7, CV-14, KI-3
Heart Yang Depletion	Warm and free heart yang	HT-5, SI-4, BL-15
	Nourish the heart and quiet the spirit	HT-7, CV-14, KI-3
	In serious cases, salvage yang and secure against desertion	CV-4†, CV-6†, ST-36†, CV-8† (on salt)
Heart Blood Depletion	Supplement blood, reinforce qi	SP-6, CV-6†
	Nourish the heart and quiet the spirit	HT-7, CV-14, KI-3
Heart Yin Depletion	Enrich yin	KI-3, SP-6
	Quiet the heart and spirit	HT-7, KI-3, CV-14

Heart Illness Patterns *(Repletion)*		
Pattern Type	Method of Treatment	Representative Points
Upflaming of Heart Fire	Drain heart fire	HT-8, BL-15
	Enrich yin and downbear fire	KI-6, SP-6, PC-8, LV-2
Cardiac Bi	Quicken the blood and transform stasis	PC-6, SP-4, SP-8, SP-10

Lung Illness Patterns		
Pattern Type	Method of Treatment	Representative Points
Non-Diffusion of Lung Qi	Diffuse the lung	LU-7, LU-1, CV-17, BL-13
Impaired Depurative Downbearing of Lung Qi	Depurate and downbear lung qi	LU-7, LU-5, KI-6
Lung Qi Depletion	Supplement yang qi in the lung	LI-4, LU-9, GV-12, BL-13
Lung Yin Depletion	Enrich yin and moisten the lung	LU-9, LU-5, KI-3, KI-10

Splenic Illness Patterns *Splenic Transformation Failure*		
Pattern Type	**Method of Treatment**	**Representative Points**
Spleen Qi Depletion	Fortify the spleen and reinforce qi	LU-9, SP-2, SP-3, BL-13, BL-20†
Devitalization of Splenic Yang	Warm yang and reinforce movement	ST-36†, SP-3†, BL-20†
Center Qi Fall	Fortify the spleen	LV-13†, BL-20†
	Upbear yang and reinforce qi	CV-6†, CV-12†, ST-30

Spleen / Stomach Illness Patterns		
Pattern Type	**Method of Treatment**	**Representative Points**
Blood Management Failure	Reinforce the qi and contain the blood	CV-6†, SP-1†, LV-1†
	Warm the spleen	BL-20†, LV-13†
Gastric Qi Depletion Cold	Fortify the center and warm the stomach	CV-12†, BL-20†, BL-21†, ST-36
Insufficiency of Stomach Yin	Nourish stomach yin	SP-4, ST-42, CV-12

Liver Illness Patterns		
Binding Depression of Liver Qi		
Pattern Type	Method of Treatment	Representative Points
General Binding Depression of Liver Qi	Course the liver and rectify qi	LI-4, LV-3, LV-14, GB-34
Invasion of the Stomach by Liver Qi	Course the liver and harmonize the stomach	LV-2, LV-3, CV-12, BL-21
Hepatosplenic Disharmony	Harmonize the liver and the spleen	BL-18, BL-20, LV-14, LV-13
Plumstone Globus	Downbear qi and transform phlegm	LU-7, ST-36, ST-40, SP-3

Liver Illness Patterns		
Ascendant and Upflaming		
Pattern Type	Method of Treatment	Representative Points
Upflaming of Liver Fire	Clear the liver and drain fire	BL-18, LV-14, LV-2, GB-34
Ascendant Hyperactivity of Liver Yang	Enrich yin and calm the liver	KI-3, KI-10, LV-2, LV-3

Liver Illness Patterns *Wind Related*		
Pattern Type	**Method of Treatment**	**Representative Points**
Liver Wind	Calm the liver and extinguish wind	LV-14, BL-18, LV-3, GB-20
Liver Blood Depletion	Nourish liver blood	LV-3, LV-14
	Enrich kidney yin	KI-3, KI-10

Kidney Illness Patterns *Yin Depletion*		
Pattern Type	**Method of Treatment**	**Representative Points**
Kidney Yin Depletion	Enrich the kidney and nourish yin	KI-3, KI-10, GB-25
Cardiorenal Yin Depletion	Enrich the kidney and nourish the heart	KI-3, KI-10, HT-7, HT-3
Hepatorenal Yin Depletion	Enrich the kidney and calm the liver	KI-3, KI-7, LV-2, LV-3
Pulmorenal Yin Depletion	Enrich the kidney and nourish the lung	KI-3, KI-7, LU-9, LU-5

Kidney Illness Patterns *Yang Depletion*		
Pattern Type	**Method of Treatment**	**Representative Points**
Kidney Yang Depletion	Warm the kidney and restore yang	KI-7†, BL-23†, GV-4†
Splenorenal Yang Depletion	Warm and supplement the spleen and kidney	BL-20†, BL-23†, SP-3†, KI-3†
Qi Absorption Failure	Warm the kidney and promote qi absorption	GV-4†, BL-23†, LU-9, CV-17
Cardiorenal Yang Debilitation	Salvage yang and secure against desertion	CV-4†, CV-6†, CV-8† (on salt)
Yang Depletion Water Flood	Warm yang and disinhibit water	GV-4†, BL-23†, SP-9, CV-9
Insufficiency of Kidney Essence	Supplement the kidney and reinforce essence	GV-4, BL-23, KI-3, CV-4
Insecurity of Kidney Qi	Secure the kidney and astringe essence	GV-4†, BL-23†, CV-4†

Stomach Illness Patterns *Counterflow Ascent of Stomach Qi*		
Pattern Type	**Method of Treatment**	**Representative Points**
Stomach Cold	Warm the stomach and dissipate cold	CV-12†, BL-21†, ST-36†, ST-41†
Stomach Heat	Drain stomach fire	BL-21, CV-12, ST-44, SP-3
Stomach Yin Insufficiency	Enrich yin and nourish the stomach	SP-4, ST-42, CV-12
Epigastric Food Stagnation	Disperse food and abduct stagnation	ST-25, CV-10
	Disinhibit the *fu* organs and drain repletion	CV-12, ST-36, ST-45
Stomach Qi Depletion	Reinforce qi and fortify the stomach and spleen	ST-36, ST-41, SP-2, SP-3, BL-20, BL-21

Large Intestine Illness Patterns		
Pattern Type	**Method of Treatment**	**Representative Points**
Large Intestine Repletion Heat (Intestinal Heat Bind)	Clear heat and abduct stagnation	LI-2, LI-11, ST-25, ST-44
Large Intestine Damp Heat	Clear heat and transform damp to stop diarrhea	ST-25, ST-36, SP-2, SP-3
Large Intestine Fluid Depletion	Enrich yin and nourish fluids	KI-3, KI-7
	Moisten the intestines and disinhibit the stool	TB-6, KI-6
Intestinal Depletion Efflux Desertion	Strengthen the intestines to secure their containment ability	LI-11†, BL-25†, ST-25†, ST-36†
Large Intestine Depletion Cold	Dissipate cold to check diarrhea	LI-11†, BL-25†, ST-25†

Small Intestine Illness Patterns		
Pattern Type	Method of Treatment	Representative Points
Depletion Cold of the Small Intestine	Warm and free the small intestine	CV-4†, BL-27†, ST-39†
Repletion Heat of the Small Intestine	Clear and disinhibit repletion heat	SI-2, BL-27, CV-4, BL-66
Small Intestine Qi Pain (Repletion Cold)	Move and dissipate binding	SI-1, SI-6, LI-9, ST-39

Gallbladder Illness Patterns		
Pattern Type	Method of Treatment	Representative Points
Gallbladder Repletion	Clear heat and disinhibit the gallbladder	BL-19, GB-24, GB-34, GB-43
Gallbladder Depletion	Clear heat and transform phlegm	BL-19, BL-20
	Downbear counter-flow and harmonize the stomach	CV-12, GB-34

Bladder Illness Patterns		
Pattern Type	Method of Treatment	Representative Points
Bladder Damp-Heat	Clear heat, dissipate damp	BL-28, CV-3, BL-40, BL-66
Bladder Depletion Cold	Secure containment of kidney qi	CV-3†, BL-23†, BL-28†

4 Treatment of Pathogen Patterns

—Overview— Pathogen Patterns	
Pathogen	**Potential Illness Pattern**
Wind	Contraction of Exogenous Wind Invasion of the Channels by the Wind Pathogen Wind-Cold-Damp *Bi*
Cold	Contraction of the Cold Pathogen Cold *Bi* Cold Pain Cold Diarrhea Cold *Shan*
Heat and Fire	Repletion Heat Depletion Heat
Summerheat	Summerheat Heat Summerheat Damp
Damp	Damp Obstruction Damp-Heat Lodged in the Qi Aspect (in Triple Burner) Splenogastric Damp Obstruction Brewing Hepatocystic Damp-Heat Downpour of Damp-Heat into the Large Intestine Downpour of Damp-Heat into the Bladder
Dryness	Contraction of Exogenous Dryness Damage to Liquid Damage to Yin Blood Dryness

(Continued)

Pathogen Patterns	
(Continued)	
Pathogen	**Potential Illness Pattern**
Phlegm	Damp Phlegm Cold Phlegm Heat Phlegm Wind-Phlegm Phlegm Confounding the Cardiac Portals Phlegm Lodging in the Channels or Limbs Phlegm Lodging in the Chest and Hypochondrium
Digestate Accumulation	Ingesta Damage Gastrointestinal Accumulation Splenic Depletion with Ingesta Damage Complication

Wind Illness Patterns		
Contraction of Exogenous Wind		
Pattern Type	**Method of Treatment**	**Representative Points**
Wind Cold	Resolve cold and exterior wind	LI-4†, TB-5†, GB-20, GV-16
Wind Heat	Clear heat and expel wind	LI-4, LI-11, GB-20, GV-16
Invasion of the Channels by the Wind Pathogen		
Local Sinews and Vessels	Dispel wind and settle tetany	Drain local *ashi*; needle *jing-well*, and supplement *yuan-source* of associated channels.
General Sinews and Vessels	Dispel wind and settle tetany	TB-5, GB-20, GV-16, BL-12, GB-34, LV-3
Wind Cold Damp Bi	Dispel wind, transform damp, and dissipate cold	Drain local points of affected channels and muscles; moxa supplementation and *yuan-source* points of associated channels

Cold Illness Patterns		
Pattern Type	Method of Treatment	Representative Points
Contraction of the Cold Pathogen	Resolve the exterior	LU-7, LI-4, TB-5, BL-12, GV-14
Cold Bi	Warm the channels and dissipate cold	LI-4†, GV-14†, ST-36†; drain local points on muscles and joints
Cold Pain	Dissipate cold and relieve abdominal pain	CV-12†, CV-6†, ST-25†, ST-36†
Cold Diarrhea	Warm the center and fortify the spleen	BL-20†, BL-21†, ST-36†, SP-2†, SP-3†
Cold Shan	Warm the liver and dissipate cold	LV-8†, BL-18†
	Rectify qi and relieve pain	LI-4, LV-3

Heat and Fire Illness Patterns		
Pattern Type	**Method of Treatment**	**Representative Points**
Repletion Heat	Clear heat and detoxify	CV-12, ST-25, ST-44
	Drain fire	M-UE-1-10 (bleed), KI-1
Depletion Heat	Enrich yin	KI-3, SP-6
	Clear heat	LI-11, BL-40

Summerheat Patterns		
Pattern Type	**Method of Treatment**	**Representative Points**
Summerheat Heat	Clear summerheat	LI-4, LI-11, GV-14, BL-40
Summerheat Damp	Clear summerheat and transform damp	LI-11, GV-14, ST-40, SP-3

Damp Illness Patterns		
Pattern Type	Method of Treatment	Representative Points
Damp Obstruction	Transform damp	ST-40, SP-3, SP-9
	Dry damp	BL-20†, LV-13†
	Disinhibit damp	SP-2, SP-3
Damp-Heat Lodged in the Qi Aspect (in Triple Burner)	Clear heat and transform damp	BL-20, BL-21, SP-9, ST-44
Splenogastric Damp Obstruction	Harmonize spleen and stomach, and move obstruction	BL-20, LV-13, BL-21, CV-12 ST-36, ST-45
Brewing Hepatocystic Damp-Heat	Course hepatocystic damp-heat	BL-18, BL-19, GB-34, LV-3
Downpour of Damp-Heat into the Large Intestine	Clear heat and disinhibit damp	LI-2, LI-11, ST-36, ST-37, SP-9
Downpour of Damp-Heat into the Bladder	Clear heat and disinhibit water	BL-28, BL-40, BL-58, KI-3, KI-7

Dryness Illness Patterns		
Pattern Type	Method of Treatment	Representative Points
Contraction of Exogenous Dryness	Clear the lung and moisten dryness	LU-7, LU-5, KI-6, KI-10
Damage to Liquid	Engender liquid and clear heat	LU-9, LI-11, KI-3, BL-40
Damage to Yin	Enrich yin humor	KI-3, LV-3, SP-6
Blood Dryness	Nourish the blood to moisten dryness	BL-20, BL-21, SP-6, ST-36

Phlegm Illness Patterns		
Pattern Type	Method of Treatment	Representative Points
Damp Phlegm	Dry damp to transform phlegm	ST-40, SP-3, SP-2†, BL-20†
Cold Phlegm	Warm and transform cold phlegm	SP-2†, SP-3†, LU-9†, ST-40
Heat Phlegm	Clear heat and transform phlegm	LI-11, ST-36, ST-40, SP-3
Wind Phlegm	Dispel wind phlegm	LV-2, LV-3, SP-2, SP-3
Upper-Body Harassment by Phlegm Turbidity	Transform phlegm and fortify the spleen	SP-2, SP-3, BL-20
	Calm the liver and extinguish wind	LV-2, BL-18, LV-14
Phlegm Confounding the Cardiac Portals	Sweep phlegm and open the portals	PC-9, GV-26, HT-7, KI-3
Phlegm Lodging in the Channels or Limbs	Disperse phlegm and soften hardness	ST-40, SP-3
	Free the connecting channels	LI-10, ST-36, local points
Phlegm Lodging in the Chest and Hypochondrium	Transform rheum and expel phlegm	PC-5, CV-22, CV-17, SP-21

Digestate Accumulation Patterns		
Pattern Type	Method of Treatment	Representative Points
Ingesta Damage	Abduct and disperse digestate	PC-6, CV-12, ST-36
Gastro-intestinal Accumulation	Promote precipitation	CV-12, ST-25, ST-37
Splenic Depletion with Ingesta Damage Complication	Increase appetite and fortify the spleen	Supplement SP-2, SP-3, BL-20; disperse ST-36, ST-37, ST-39

5 Treatment of Exogenous Heat Patterns

—Overview— Exogenous Heat Patterns	
Six-Channel Patterns	Taiyang, Yangming, Shaoyang, Taiyin, Shaoyin, Jueyin
Four-Aspect Patterns	Defense (*wei*), Qi, Construction (*ying*), Blood
Triple-Burner Patterns	Upper Burner (Lung and Pericardium) Middle Burner (Stomach and Spleen) Lower Burner (Liver and Kidney)
Pericardiac Patterns	Inward Fall of Pathogens to the Pericardium Clouding of the Pericardium by Phlegm Turbidity Stomach Heat Sweltering the Pericardium

5.1 Treatment of Six-Channel Patterns (The Cold Damage School)

—Overview— Six-Channel Patterns		
Pattern	**Pathomechanism**	**Manifestations**
Taiyang	Assailment of the exterior by wind cold	Exterior Repletion Exterior Depletion
Yangming	Gastrointestinal repletion heat	Channel Pattern Bowel Pattern
Shaoyang	Pathogen at midstage between exterior and interior	Exterior Pattern Interior Pattern
Taiyin	Gastrointestinal depletion cold	Like *yangming* bowel pattern but with signs of depletion
Shaoyin	Cardiorenal debilitation	Depletion Cold Depletion Heat
Jueyin	Interior depletion and cold/heat complex	Upper body heat with lower body cold

Taiyang Illness Patterns		
Patho-mechanism	**Method of Treatment**	**Representative Points**
Assailment of the exterior by wind-cold	Resolve the exterior and dissipate wind	LU-7, LI-4, TB-5, GB-20, GV-16, BL-12

Yangming Illness Patterns			
Patho-mechanism		**Method of Treatment**	**Representative Points**
Gastrointestinal repletion heat	*Channel Pattern*	Clear heat from the yangming channel	LI-3, LI-4, LI-11, ST-44, ST-41
	Bowel Pattern	Promote precipitation	LI-11, ST-25, left SP-13, ST-36

Shaoyang Illness Patterns		
Patho-mechanism	**Method of Treatment**	**Representative Points**
Pathogen at midstage between exterior and interior	Harmonize the exterior and interior	TB-3, GB-41, LV-14, PC-5, GB-44, CV-12

Taiyin Illness Patterns		
Patho-mechanism	Method of Treatment	Representative Points
Gastrosplenic depletion cold	Warm the center and fortify the spleen	SP-1†, SP-4†, SP-6†, CV-12†, LV-13†

Shaoyin Illness Patterns			
Patho-mechanism	Differentiation	Method of Treatment	Representative Points
Cardiorenal debilitation	Depletion cold	Salvage yang and check counter-flow	GV-4†, CV-6†, ST-36†
	Depletion heat	Enrich yin to clear heat	BL-23, CV-4, KI-3, KI-7

Jueyin Illness Patterns		
Patho-mechanism	Method of Treatment	Representative Points
Interior depletion and cold-heat complex	Pure yang pattern	LV-1, LV-4, HT-4, BL-18,
	Pure yin pattern	BL-18†, LV-2†, CV-4†, CV-12†, LV-14†
	Mixed yin/yang pattern	LV-4, HT-4, CV-4†, PC-5†, BL-18

5.2 Treatment of Four-Aspect Patterns (The Thermic-Illness School)

—Overview— Four-Aspect Patterns		
Pattern	**Pathomechanism**	**Differentiation**
Defense	Pathogen in the defensive exterior	Wind Thermia Damp Thermia
Qi	Exuberant heat in the qi aspect	First Stage Qi Aspect Heat Exuberant Pulmogastric Heat Great Heat in the Qi Aspect Gastrointestinal Heat Bind Heat Lodging in the Triple Burner Brewing Damp-Heat Steaming the Intestines and Stomach
Construction	Inward fall of pathogenic heat to the construction aspect	Inward Fall of Thermic Heat or Wind Thermia Inward Fall of Damp Thermia
Blood	Penetration of pathogenic heat to the blood aspect, causing depletion or frenetic blood movement	Repletion Heat at the Blood Aspect Depletion Heat at the Blood Aspect

Defense Aspect Illness Patterns		
Pathogen in the defensive exterior		
Differentiation	**Method of Treatment**	**Representative Points**
Wind Thermia	Expel wind from the exterior	LI-4, TB-3, LU-10, BL-12, BL-13
Damp Thermia	Promote diffusion and transformation	LU-7, LI-4, PC-6, CV-13, CV-12, ST-44

Qi Aspect Illness Patterns		
Exuberant heat in the qi aspect		
Differentiation	**Method of Treatment**	**Representative Points**
First Stage Qi Aspect Heat	Clear and outthrust pathogenic heat	TB-2, TB-3, PC-7
Exuberant Pulmogastric Heat	Clear heat and diffuse the lung	LU-10, LU-11, LI-2, LI-11, BL-13, BL-21
Great Heat in the Qi Aspect	Drain heat	LU-10, LI-4, TB-2, GV-14, BL-13, ST-36, ST-44
Gastrointestinal Heat Bind	Flush accumulated heat	CV-12, ST-25, BL-20, BL-21, ST-36, BL-40, ST-44
Heat Lodging in the Triple Burner	Transform phlegm and clear heat	PC-6, CV-12, ST-36, ST-40, SP-3
Brewing Damp-Heat Steaming the Intestine and Stomach	Dry damp and drain heat	ST-25, ST-36, ST-44, BL-21, BL-25, SP-2, SP-3

Construction Aspect Illness Patterns	
Inward Fall of pathogenic heat to the construction aspect	
Method of Treatment	**Representative Points**
Clear heat from the construction aspect	BL-15, BL-18, BL-20, BL-23, LU-5, HT-7, KI-3

Blood Aspect Illness Patterns	
Penetration of pathogenic heat to blood aspect causing depletion or frenetic movement of the blood	
Method of Treatment	**Representative Points**
Cool the blood and resolve toxin	SP-6, SP-10, BL-40, PC-5, HT-3

5.3 Treatment of Triple Burner Penetration

Triple Burner Pathogen Penetration		
Upper Burner		
Lung	Clear pathogenic heat from the lungs, moisten lung dryness	LU-7, LU-5, BL-12, BL-13, CV-17, KI-6
Pericardium	Clear pathogenic heat from thorax, moisten dryness	PC-6, PC-3, BL-14, BL-15, CV-14, SP-4
Middle Burner		
Stomach	Clear stomach heat, moisten dryness	BL-21, BL-22, TB-6, CV-12, ST-36, ST-44
Spleen	Clear splenic heat, dry damp	BL-20, LV-13, SP-2, SP-9
Lower Burner		
Kidney	Nourish kidney yin	LU-9, LU-5, KI-3, KI-10, CV-4
Liver	Subdue liver yang	LV-2, LV-3, LV-14, GB-34, GB-43, BL-18, BL-19

5.4 Treatment of Pericardiac Patterns

Pericardiac Patterns		
Patho-mechanism	Method of Treatment	Representative Points
Inward fall of thermic pathogens to the pericardium	Open the cardiac portals, drain pathogenic heat	PC-9, HT-9, GV-26, KI-1
Clouding of the pericardium by phlegm turbidity	Open the cardiac portals, salvage yang	PC-9, HT-9, CV-4†, CV-6†, CV-8† (on salt)
Stomach heat sweltering the pericardium	Precipitate gastrointestinal heat	LI-1, LI-11, BL-21, BL-22, BL-25, ST-36, ST-45

6 Channel Depletion and Repletion: Five-Phase Treatment Approaches

Use of Transporting-*shu* Points			
Channel Condition		Treatment via Affected Channel	Treatment via Mother or Child Channel
Lung	Depletion	LU-9, earth of metal channel	SP-3, earth of earth channel
	Repletion	LU-5, water of metal channel	KI-10, water of water channel
Heart	Depletion	HT-9, wood of fire channel	LV-1, wood of wood channel
	Repletion	HT-7, earth of fire channel	SP-3, earth of earth channel
Pericardium	Depletion	PC-9, wood of fire channel	LV-1, wood of wood channel
	Repletion	PC-7, earth of fire channel	SP-3, earth of earth channel
Large Intestine	Depletion	LI-11, earth of metal channel	ST-36, earth of earth channel
	Repletion	LI-2, water of metal channel	BL-66, water of water channel
Small Intestine	Depletion	SI-3, wood of fire channel	GB-41, wood of wood channel
	Repletion	SI-8, earth of fire channel	ST-36, earth of earth channel
Triple Burner	Depletion	TB-3, wood of fire channel	GB-41, wood of wood channel
	Repletion	TB-10, earth of fire channel	ST-36, earth of earth channel
Spleen	Depletion	SP-2, fire of earth channel	HT-8, fire of fire channel
	Repletion	SP-5, metal of earth channel	LU-8, metal of metal channel
Kidney	Depletion	KI-7, metal of water channel	LU-8, metal of metal channel
	Repletion	KI-1, wood of water channel	LV-1, wood of wood channel
Liver	Depletion	LV-8, water of wood channel	KI-10, water of water channel
	Repletion	LV-2, fire of wood channel	HT-8, fire of fire channel
Stomach	Depletion	ST-41, fire of earth channel	SI-5, fire of fire channel
	Repletion	ST-45, metal of earth channel	LI-1, metal of metal channel
Bladder	Depletion	BL-67, metal of water channel	LI-1, metal of metal channel
	Repletion	BL-65, wood of water channel	GB-41, wood of wood channel
Gallbladder	Depletion	GB-43, water of wood channel	BL-66, water of water channel
	Repletion	GB-38, fire of wood channel	SI-5, fire of fire channel

Channel	Depletion Patterns				Repletion Patterns			
	Supplement		*Drain*		Supplement		*Drain*	
LU	**SP-3**	**LU-9**	*HT-8*	*LU-10*	**HT-8**	**LU-10**	*KI-10*	*LU-5*
LI	**ST-36**	**LI-11**	*SI-5*	*LI-5*	**SI-5**	**LI-5**	*BL-66*	*LI-2*
ST	**SI-5**	**ST-41**	*GB-41*	*ST-43*	**GB-41**	**ST-43**	*LI-1*	*ST-45*
SP	**HT-8**	**SP-2**	*LV-1*	*SP-1*	**LV-1**	**SP-1**	*LU-8*	*SP-5*
HT	**LV-1**	**HT-9**	*KI-10*	*HT-3*	**KI-10**	**HT-3**	*SP-3*	*HT-7*
SI	**GB-41**	**SI-3**	*BL-66*	*SI-2*	**BL-66**	**SI-2**	*ST-36*	*SI-8*
BL	**LI-1**	**BL-67**	*ST-36*	*BL-40*	**ST-36**	**BL-40**	*GB-41*	*BL-65*
KI	**LU-8**	**KI-7**	*SP-3*	*KI-3*	**SP-3**	**KI-3**	*LV-1*	*KI-1*
PC	**LV-1**	**PC-9**	*KI-10*	*PC-3*	**KI-10**	**PC-3**	*SP-3*	*PC-7*
TB	**GB-41**	**TB-3**	*BL-66*	*TB-2*	**BL-66**	**TB-2**	*ST-36*	*TB-10*
GB	**BL-66**	**GB-43**	*LI-1*	*GB-44*	**LI-1**	**GB-44**	*SI-5*	*GB-38*
LV	**KI-10**	**LV-8**	*LU-8*	*LV-4*	**LU-8**	**LV-4**	*HT-8*	*LV-2*

Korean Four-Point Five-Phase Treatments
Depletion and Repletion Patterns

Korean Four-Point Five-Phase Treatments *Cold and Heat Patterns*							
Channel	Cold Patterns				Heat Patterns		
	Supplement		*Drain*		Supplement		*Drain*
LU	**HT-8**	**LU-10**	*LU-5*	*KI-10*	**LU-5**	**KI-10**	*SP-3*	*LU-9*
LI	**SI-5**	**ST-41**	*LI-2*	*BL-66*	**LI-2**	**BL-66**	*SI-5*	*ST-41*
ST	**ST-41**	**SI-5**	*ST-44*	*BL-66*	**ST-44**	**BL-66**	*ST-36*	*BL-40*
SP	**SP-2**	**HT-8**	*SP-9*	*KI-10*	**SP-9**	**KI-10**	*SP-3*	*KI-3*
HT	**HT-8**	**KI-2**	*HT-3*	*KI-10*	**HT-3**	**KI-10**	*HT-8*	*KI-2*
SI	**SI-5**	**BL-60**	*SI-2*	*BL-66*	**SI-2**	**BL-66**	*SI-8*	*ST-36*
BL	**SI-5**	**BL-60**	*SI-2*	*BL-66*	**SI-2**	**BL-66**	*ST-36*	*BL-40*
KI	**HT-8**	**KI-2**	*KI-10*	*HT-3*	**KI-10**	**HT-3**	*SP-3*	*KI-3*
PC	**HT-8**	**PC-8**	*PC-3*	*HT-3*	**PC-3**	**HT-3**	*SP-3*	*PC-7*
TB	**TB-6**	**BL-60**	*TB-2*	*BL-66*	**TB-2**	**BL-66**	*TB-6*	*BL-60*
GB	**GB-38**	**SI-5**	*GB-43*	*BL-66*	**GB-43**	**BL-66**	*BL-40*	*GB-34*
LV	**LV-2**	**HT-8**	*KI-10*	*LV-8*	**KI-10**	**LV-8**	*LV-3*	*SP-3*

Chinese Six-Point Five-Phase Treatments *Depletion Patterns*							
Depleted Phase		**Supplement**		*Drain*			
Wood		**Water**		*Metal*		*Earth*	
	LV	**LV-8**	**KI-10**	*LV-4*	*LU-8*	*LV-3*	*SP-3*
	GB	**GB-43**	**BL-66**	*GB-44*	*LI-1*	*GB-34*	*ST-36*
Fire		**Wood**		*Water*		*Metal*	
	HT	**HT-9**	**LV-1**	*HT-3*	*KI-10*	*HT-4*	*LU-8*
	SI	**SI-3**	**GB-41**	*SI 2*	*BL-66*	*SI-1*	*LI-1*
Earth		**Fire**		*Wood*		*Water*	
	SP	**SP-2**	**HT-8**	*SP-1*	*LV-1*	*SP-9*	*KI-10*
	ST	**ST-41**	**SI-5**	*ST-43*	*GB-41*	*ST-44*	*BL-66*
Metal		**Earth**		*Fire*		*Wood*	
	LU	**LU-9**	**SP-3**	*LU-10*	*HT-8*	*LU-11*	*LV-1*
	LI	**LI-11**	**ST-36**	*LI-5*	*SI-5*	*LI-3*	*GB-41*
Water		**Metal**		*Earth*		*Fire*	
	KI	**KI-7**	**LU-8**	*KI-3*	*SP-3*	*KI-2*	*HT-8*
	BL	**BL-67**	**LI-1**	*BL-40*	*ST-36*	*BL-60*	*SI-5*
Fire (Ministerial)		**Wood**		*Water*		*Metal*	
	PC	**PC-9**	**LV-1**	*PC-3*	*KI-10*	*PC-5*	*LU-8*
	TB	**TB-3**	**GB-41**	*TB-2*	*BL-66*	*TB-1*	*ST-45*

Chinese Six-Point Five-Phase Treatments *Repletion Patterns*								
Replete Phase		*Drain*		Supplement				
Wood		*Fire*		**Metal**		**Earth**		
	LV	*LV-2*	*HT-8*	**LV-4**	**LU-8**	**LV-3**	**SP-3**	
	GB	*GB-38*	*SI-5*	**GB-44**	**LI-1**	**GB-34**	**ST-36**	
Fire		*Earth*		**Water**		**Metal**		
	HT	*HT-7*	*SP-3*	**HT-3**	**KI-10**	**HT-4**	**LU-8**	
	SI	*SI-8*	*ST-36*	**SI-2**	**BL-66**	**SI-1**	**LI-1**	
Earth		*Metal*		**Wood**		**Water**		
	SP	*SP-5*	*LU-8*	**SP-1**	**LV-1**	**SP-9**	**KI-10**	
	ST	*ST-45*	*LI-1*	**ST-43**	**GB-41**	**ST-44**	**BL-66**	
Metal		*Water*		**Fire**		**Wood**		
	LU	*LU-5*	*KI-10*	**LU-10**	**HT-8**	**LU-11**	**LV-1**	
	LI	*LI-2*	*BL-66*	**LI-5**	**SI-5**	**LI-3**	**GB-41**	
Water		*Wood*		**Earth**		**Fire**		
	KI	*KI-1*	*LV-1*	**KI-3**	**SP-3**	**KI-2**	**HT-8**	
	BL	*BL-65*	*GB-41*	**BL-40**	**ST-36**	**BL-60**	**SI-5**	
Fire (Ministerial)		*Earth*		**Water**		**Metal**		
	PC	*PC-7*	*SP-3*	**PC-3**	**KI-10**	**PC-5**	**LU-8**	
	TB	*TB-10*	*ST-36*	**TB-2**	**BL-66**	**TB-1**	**ST-45**	

North-South Point Selection				
Disease Pattern	**Distinguishing Characteristics**	**Treatment Principle**	**Points Selected**	
			Yin Channels	Yang Channels
Liver repletion with Lung depletion	Spleen (earth) remains unaffected	Supplement water on water channels	KI-10 KI-7	BL-66 BL-67
		Drain fire on fire channels	HT-8 HT-7	SI-5 SI-8
Heart repletion with Kidney depletion	Lung (metal) remains unaffected	Supplement wood on wood channels	LV-1 LV-8	GB-41 GB-43
		Drain earth on earth channels	SP-3 SP-5	ST-36 ST-45
Spleen repletion with Liver depletion	Kidney (water) remains unaffected	Supplement fire on fire channels	HT-8 HT-9	SI-5 SI-3
		Drain metal on metal channels	LU-8 LU-5	LI-1 LI-2
Liver repletion with Heart depletion	Liver (wood) remains unaffected	Supplement earth on earth channels	SP-3 SP-2	ST-36 ST-41
		Drain water on water channels	KI-10 KI-1	BL-66 BL-65
Kidney repletion with Spleen depletion	Heart (fire) remains unaffected	Supplement metal on metal channels	LU-8 LU-9	LI-1 LI-11
		Drain wood on wood channels	LV-1 LV-2	GB-41 GB-38

Part II

Illustrative
Treatments

7 Selected Gastrointestinal Disorders

Abdominal Pain	
Cold Accumulation	
Symptoms:	Sudden onset, violent pain that responds to warmth and is exacerbated by cold, loose stool, absence of thirst, clear, profuse urine, cold limbs
Pulse:	Deep and tense, or deep and slow *Tongue:* thin, white fur
Treatment:	Warm middle burner: **CV-12†, CV-8†** (on salt) Strengthen splenogastric function: **SP-4†, ST-36†**
Splenic Yang Depletion	
Symptoms:	Intermittent, dull pain, relieved by warmth or pressure, exacerbated by cold or hunger; lassitude, loose stool
Pulse:	Deep, thready
Tongue:	Thin, white coating
Treatment:	Supplement spleen and stomach yang: **BL-20†, BL-21†, CV-12†, LV-13†** Supplement qi: **CV-6†, ST-36†**
Food Retention	
Symptoms:	Distention and pain in epigastrium and abdomen which is aggravated by pressure, anorexia, foul belching, sour regurgitation; abdominal pain accompanied by diarrhea and relieved after defecation
Pulse:	Rolling
Tongue:	Sticky coating
Treatment:	Promote descent of stomach qi: **CV-12, ST-36** Regulate intestines: **CV-6, ST-25** Calm the stomach and relieve stagnation: **ST-44**
Treatment by affected area:	Pain above umbilicus: **SP-4, CV-10, ST-24** Pain around umbilicus: **KI-5, CV-6, ST-25** Pain below umbilicus: **SP-6, CV-4, ST-29**

Epigastric Pain
Food Retention

Symptoms:	Distention and pain in epigastrium which is worse after eating, pain aggravated by pressure, fetid belching, anorexia
Pulse:	Deep, forceful, rolling
Tongue:	Thick, sticky coating
Treatment:	Relieve epigastric fullness: **PC-6, ST-44** Promote descending function of stomach: **CV-12, ST-36** Fortify spleen to promote digestion: **LV-13**

Invasion of Stomach by Liver Qi

Symptoms:	Paroxysmal epigastric pain, distention and pain in hypochondrium, nausea, abdominal distention, acid upflow, frequent belching, anorexia
Pulse:	Deep, wiry
Tongue:	Thin, white coating
Treatment:	Harmonize liver qi: **LV-3, LV-14** Calm middle burner, relieve nausea, promote descent: **PC-6, CV-12, ST-36**

Stomach Depletion with Cold Stagnation

Symptoms:	Dull pain in epigastrium, general lassitude, regurgitation of thin fluid, pain alleviated by warmth or pressure
Pulse:	Deep, slow
Tongue:	Thin, white coating
Treatment:	Regulate middle burner: **PC-6, SP-4** Warm middle burner: **CV-12†** Dispel cold: **CV-6** (ginger moxibustion) Fortify spleen and stomach: **ST-36†, BL-20†**

Hypochondriac Pain

General Treatment:	Regulate qi in shaoyang channels: **TB-6, GB-34** Relieve pain in hypochondrium: **LV-14**

Repletion Patterns

Qi Stagnation

Symptoms:	Distending pain in costal and hyponchondriac regions, fullness in chest, sighing, bitter taste in mouth, poor appetite
Pulse:	Wiry *Tongue:* Thin, white coating
Treatment:	Promote liver-gallbladder function of maintaining patency of qi flow: **LV-3, BL-18, GB-40**

Blood Stasis

Symptoms:	Fixed, stabbing pain in hypochondriac region, intensified by pressure and at night
Pulse:	Deep, hesitant *Tongue:* Dark purple body, or petechiae
Treatment:	Activate blood circulation, relieve stasis: **BL-17, BL-18, SP-6**

Depletion Patterns

Symptoms:	Dull, lingering pain in costal and hypochondriac region, dry mouth, irritability, dizziness, blurred vision
Pulse:	Weak, rapid, or thready *Tongue:* Red body, little or no coating
Treatment:	Nourish blood: **LV-3, LV-14, BL-18** Reinforce essence: **BL-23** Supplement gastrosplenic function: **SP-6, ST-36**

Stomach Hyperacidity

General Symptoms:	Severe stomach pains with unsettled spirit, poor appetite, gradual upflooding of sour fluid into the throat, eructation, and cardialgia. Symptoms often start two hours after eating. Pain may radiate to the shoulders.
Treatment:	Calm the liver: **BL-18, BL-17** Regulate the stomach: **BL-21, CV-12** Check stomach pain: **ST-34**

Chronic Gastritis - Stomach Cold

Symptoms:	Irregular stomach pains, sometimes light, sometimes heavy. Discomfort after meals, exacerbated by cold food. Heart palpitations, gurgling sounds in the stomach, expectoration of frothy saliva; if extreme, foul breath, clamoring stomach, sour expectoration, false sensations of hunger, epigastric distress.
Pulse:	Tight
Tongue:	Unclean fur
Treatment:	Regulate gastrointestinal secretions: **CV-12†, ST-36†** Regulate digestion: **BL-18†, BL-21†, CV-13†** Quell stomach pains: **PC-6, SP-4**

Acute Gastritis

General Symptoms:	Aversion to food, thoracic oppression, nausea and vomiting, thirst, gripping pains in the stomach and intestines, foul or rotten-smelling eructation, constipation or diarrhea; in extreme cases, headache and fever.
Pulse:	Slippery, rapid, or deep and bound
Tongue:	Greasy yellow fur, red body
Treatment:	Disinhibit stomach qi: **CV-12, ST-36** Downbear digestate: **BL-21, ST-25** Check stomach pain: **PC-6, SP-4** If due to food poisoning, add: **KI-9**

Stomach Upset

General Symptoms:	Uneasy or queasy sensation in the stomach, sensations as if stomach is "turning," etc.
Treatment:	Clear the stomach and downbear counterflow: Drain **CV-12, ST-25, CV-17**; *zhongkui* (**M-UE-16†**) Conduct stomach qi downwards to check vomiting: Drain **ST-36**

Abdominal Distention

General Treatment:	Relieve abdominal fullness: **CV-12, ST-36** Relieve intestinal stagnation: **ST-25, ST-37**

Repletion

Symptoms:	Abdominal pain, distention, and fullness that is aggravated by pressure, belching, foul breath, dark yellow urine, constipation; possibly fever
Pulse:	Rolling, rapid, forceful *Tongue:* Thick, yellow coating
Treatment:	Promote qi circulation to relieve fullness: **LI-4, CV-6** Drain damp heat: **SP-9**

Depletion

Symptoms:	Abdominal distention that is relieved by pressure, borborygmi, loose stools, anorexia, lassitude, listlessness, clear urine
Pulse:	Forceless *Tongue:* Pale body
Treatment:	Strengthen spleen and stomach: **SP-3†, ST-36†** Strengthen lower burner to promote intestinal function: **CV-4†**

Alimentary Tract Obstruction

Symptoms:	Poor appetite, poor digestion, followed by heavy pressure in the stomach, difficulty in swallowing food; or after swallowing food, slight agitation and a choking sensation in the chest. Symptoms all increase daily, until only liquids can be taken.
Pulse:	fine, and rough or wiry Tongue: Ashen white fur, or stagnant yellow fur
Treatment:	Downbear counterflow: Drain **CV-22, CV-17, PC-6, BL-43, GV-12, ST-36** Nourish yin: Supplement **KI-7** Regulate stomach and spleen: Drain **BL-20, BL-21**

Vomiting	
General Treatment:	Regulate middle burner: **PC-6, SP-4** Relieve central fullness: **CV-12, ST-36**
Retention of Food	
Symptoms:	Epigastric and abdominal distention or pain, acidic vomitus, belching, loose stool or constipation, anorexia, foul gas
Pulse:	Rolling, forceful
Tongue:	Thick, sticky, granular coating
Treatment:	Relieve gastric and intestinal obstruction: **CV-10, ST-25**
Invasion of the Stomach by Liver Qi	
Symptoms:	Vomiting, acid regurgitation, continual belching, irritability, distending pain in hypochondrium
Pulse:	Wiry
Tongue:	Thin, sticky coating
Treatment:	Calm liver function: **LV-3, LV-14**
Gastrosplenic Depletion	
Symptoms:	Sallow complexion, vomiting after meals, anorexia, slightly loose stools, general lassitude
Pulse:	Forceless
Tongue:	Thin white, or sticky coating
Treatment:	Fortify spleen: **BL-20†**
Persistent Vomiting	
Bleed empirical points **M-HN-20a&b** (*jinjin, yuye*)	

Diarrhea

General Treatment:	Regulate large intestine: **ST-25, BL-25** Strengthen transporting function of spleen and stomach: **ST-36**

Acute Diarrhea

Cold-Damp

Symptoms:	Watery diarrhea, abdominal pain and borborygmus, chilliness that responds to warmth, absence of thirst
Pulse:	Deep, slow *Tongue:* Pale body with white coating
Treatment:	Warm spleen and stomach to dispel damp and cold: **CV-6†, CV-12†**

Damp-Heat

Symptoms:	Diarrhea with yellow, hot, loose, fetid stools, abdominal pain, burning sensation in anus, scant dark urine; possibly fever and thirst
Pulse:	Rolling, rapid *Tongue:* Yellow, sticky coating
Treatment:	Clear intestinal dampness: **LI-4, SP-9, ST-44**

Chronic Diarrhea

Spleen Yang Depletion

Symptoms:	Loose stools with undigested food, epigastric and abdominal distention, anorexia, lassitude
Pulse:	Thready, forceless *Tongue:* Thin white coating
Treatment:	Fortify splenic yang: **BL-20†** Strengthen middle burner function: **SP-3, CV-12†, LV-13†**

Kidney Yang Depletion

Symptoms:	Slight abdominal pain, borborygmus, early morning diarrhea, chilliness in abdomen and lower extremities
Pulse:	Deep, forceless *Tongue:* White coating
Treatment:	Invigorate kidney yang: **BL-23, GV-4, KI-3** Fortify original qi: **CV-4†** Raise sunken qi of stomach and spleen: **GV-20†**

Dysentery	
General Treatment:	Supplement intestinal function: **LI-4, ST-25, ST-37**
Damp-Heat	
Symptoms:	Abdominal pain, tenesmus, mucus (usually red) in stool, burning sensation in anus, scant yellow urine; possibly chills or fever, restlessness, nausea, vomiting
Pulse:	Rolling, rapid; or soft, rapid
Tongue:	Yellow, sticky coating
Treatment:	Clear damp and heat from intestines and stomach: **LI-11, ST-44, SP-9**
Cold-Damp	
Symptoms:	Scant defecation, mainly white mucus in stool, response to warmth and aversion to cold, possibly fullness in chest and epigastrium, lingering abdominal pain, insipid taste in mouth, absence of thirst
Pulse:	Deep, slow
Tongue:	White, sticky coating
Treatment:	Warm spleen and stomach to dispel cold: **CV-6†, CV-12†** Fortify spleen to dispel damp: **SP-6**
Chronic Dysentery	
Symptoms:	Prolonged, persistent, or recurrent dysentery; possibly accompanied by lassitude, sallow complexion, chilliness, anorexia
Pulse:	Deep, thready
Tongue:	Sticky coating
Treatment:	Fortify spleen and stomach, eliminate intestinal stagnation: **BL-20†, BL-21†, CV-4†, CV-12†, ST-36†**
Treatment according to symptom:	Fever: **GV-14** Tenesmus: **BL-29** Rectal prolapse: **GV-20†, GV-1**

Constipation

General Symptoms:	Infrequent, difficult defecation, once every three to five days, or even longer in some cases.
General Treatment:	Supplement large intestine qi: **BL-25, ST-25** Clear the triple burner: **TB-6, KI-6** (this is a classical prescription for constipation)

Repletion Patterns

Heat Accumulation Constipation

Symptoms:	Constipation with fever, thirst, foul breath
Pulse:	Rolling, forceful *Tongue:* Dry, yellow coating
Treatment:	Drain *yangming* heat: **LI-4, LI-11**

Qi Stagnation Constipation

Symptoms:	Abdominal pain, fullness, and distention, frequent belching, anorexia
Pulse:	Wiry *Tongue:* Thin, sticky coating
Treatment:	Supplement qi of *fu* organs: **CV-12** Soothe liver yin to promote patent flow: **LV-3**

Depletion Patterns

Qi-Blood Depletion Constipation

Symptoms:	Pale, lusterless complexion, lips, and nails, dizziness, palpitation, shortness of breath
Pulse:	Thready, weak *Tongue:* Pale body with thin coating
Treatment:	Supplement gastrosplenic qi: **BL-20†, BL-21†, ST-36†**

Cold Accumulation Constipation

Symptoms:	Pain and cold sensation in abdomen, aversion to cold and preference for warmth
Pulse:	Deep, slow *Tongue:* Pale body with moist, white coating
Treatment:	Warm lower burner to loosen bowels: **CV6†, CV-8†** (on salt)

Rectal Prolapse	
Symptoms:	Slow onset with dragging sensation in rectum during defecation; possibly accompanied by lassitude, weakness in limbs, sallow complexion, dizziness, palpitation
Pulse:	Thready, feeble *Tongue:* Pale body with white coating
Treatment:	Raise qi in the governing vessel: **GV-20†, GV-1** Supplement large intestine qi: **BL-25†, ST-36†**

8   Selected Musculo-Skeletal Disorders

Sprain and Contusion	
General Symptoms:	Local soreness, distention, and pain; mild redness and swelling; limited or no movement
General Treatment:	Local *ashi* points plus local and distal points on related channels: Neck: **BL-10, SI-3** Shoulder: **GB-21, LI-15** Elbow: **LI-11, LI-4** Wrist: **TB-4, TB-5** Hip: **GB-30, GB-34** Knee: **ST-35, ST-44** Ankle: **ST-41, GB-40, BL-60**
Note: Needle points on the *unaffected* side first.	

Torticollis	
General Symptoms:	Wry neck caused by awkward sleeping posture, wind-cold attack, etc. Stiffness and pain of neck and nape with twisting toward one side and difficulty in flexion and extension
General Treatment:	Free circulation in local channels using local and distal points: **GV-14, BL-10, SI-14, SI-3, GB-39, BL-60** Promote circulation to aid flexion and extension: **LU-7, SI-7** Empirical point for stiff neck: **M-UE-24** (*luozhen*)

Low Back Pain	
General Treatment:	Supplement kidney qi: **BL-23†, GV-3†** Course bladder channel: **BL-40** (bleed capillaries), **BL-58**

Cold-Damp

Symptoms:	Heavy sensation and pain in dorsolumbar region, muscle stiffness, limited flexion and extension of trunk; pain may radiate down toward buttocks and lower extremities; affected area feels cold. Intensified on cloudy and rainy days; not alleviated by bedrest
Pulse:	Deep and weak, or deep and slow
Tongue:	Sticky, white coating
Treatment:	Dispel cold and damp, activate local circulation: **BL-25†, BL-26†**

Kidney Depletion Patterns

General Symptoms:	Insidious onset, protracted pain and soreness, lassitude and weakness of lumbar area and knees. Symptoms intensified after stress or strain; alleviated by bed rest.

Kidney Yang Depletion

Symptoms:	Cramping in lower abdomen, pallor, cold extremities
Pulse:	Deep and thready, or deep and slow
Tongue:	Pale body
Treatment:	Supplement kidney yang: **GV-4†, M-BW-24†** (*yaoyan*)

Kidney Yin Depletion

Symptoms:	Irritability, insomnia, dry mouth and throat, flushed face, "fever in five hearts" (heat sensation in chest, palms, and soles)
Pulse:	Weak and thready, or rapid and thready
Tongue:	Red body with little coating
Treatment:	Supplement kidney yin: **KI-3, BL-52**

(Continued)

Low Back Pain *(Continued)*	
Traumatic Injury (Lumbar Sprain, etc.)	
Symptoms:	Rigidity and pain of lower back; pain is fixed and aggravated by pressure or turning of the body
Pulse:	Wiry, hesitant
Tongue:	Pink, or dark purplish body
Treatment:	Special points for traumatic injury of the spine: **GV-26, M-UE-19** (*yao-tong*), local *ashi* points. Relieve pain and stagnation in bladder channel: **BL-40** (bleed)

9 Selected Urogenital Disorders

Dysuria (Strangury)	
General Treatment:	Supplement bladder qi: **BL-28, CV-3** Promote diuresis: **SP-9**

Dysuria Caused by Calculi (Calculous Strangury)

Symptoms:	Calculi in urine, dark yellow or turbid urine, sudden interruption of urination, lumbar and abdominal pain; possibly blood in urine
Pulse:	rapid　　　*Tongue:* normal
Treatment:	Promote flow in water passages: **BL-39**

Qi Dysfunction Dysuria (Qi Strangury)

Symptoms:	Difficult, hesitant urination, fullness and pain in lower abdomen
Pulse:	Deep, wiry　　　*Tongue:* Thin, white coating
Treatment:	Calm liver to promote patent qi flow: **LV-2**

Dysuria with Milky Urine (Unctuous Strangury)

Symptoms:	Cloudy urine, burning urethral pain during urination
Pulse:	Thready, rapid　　　*Tongue:* Red body, sticky coating
Treatment:	Reinforce kidney qi: **BL-23†, KI-6**

Overstrain Dysuria (Taxation Strangury)

Symptoms:	Difficulty in urination, intermittent dribbling of urine, usually exacerbated when fatigued, weak pulse
Treatment:	Supplement qi: **GV-20†, CV-6†, ST-36†**

Dysuria with Blood (Blood Strangury)

Symptoms:	Purplish-red streaks of blood on the urine, acute pain and distention, and heat, disfluency, and piercing pain when urinating
Pulse:	Rapid, forceful　　　*Tongue:* thin yellow fur
Treatment:	Clear heat: **BL-40, BL-66, CV-3** Cool blood: **SP-6, SP-10**

Urinary Retention

Damp-Heat Accumulation in Bladder

Symptoms:	Hot, scant urine or retention of urine, lower abdominal distention, thirst without desire to drink; possibly constipation
Pulse:	Rapid, or thready and rapid
Tongue:	Red body with yellow coating on posterior part
Treatment:	Supplement bladder qi: **BL-28, CV-3** Eliminate damp and heat: **SP-9** Promote circulation in water passages: **BL-39**

Damage to Channel Qi

Symptoms:	Dribbling urination or complete retention, distention and dull pain in lower abdomen
Pulse:	Hesitant, rapid
Tongue:	Purple petechiae
Treatment:	Regulate bladder to promote urination: **CV-3** Reinforce circulation in lower burner: **SP-6** Relieve abdominal distention and pain: **KI-5, ST-28**

Kidney yang depletion

Symptoms:	Dribbling urination that lessens in force, pallor, listlessness, chilliness and weakness in lumbar region and knee
Pulse:	Deep, thready, especially weak in proximal (third) position
Tongue:	Pale body
Treatment:	Supplement kidney yang (*mingmen*): **GV-4†, BL-23†** Strengthen kidney qi to promote urination: **CV-4†** Lift yang qi to support kidneys: **GV-20** Supplement triple burner to promote circulation in water passages: **TB-4**

Urinary Incontinence	
General Symptoms:	Loss of urinary control, particularly in older people
Pulse:	Empty, fine forceless
Tongue:	Pale body
Treatment:	Supplement lower origin qi: moxa **CV-6, CV-4, BL-23, GV-4** For nightime urination add: needle **BL-40, SP-9, SP-6**

Nocturnal Enuresis	
Symptoms:	Involuntary urination during sleep; possibly accompanied by sallow complexion, anorexia, lassitude
Pulse:	Thready, weak at proximal (third) position
Tongue:	Pale body with white coating
Treatment:	Strengthen kidneys: **Bl-23†** Regulate bladder function: **BL-28†, CV-3†** Activate foot yin channels to strengthen urogenital function: **SP-6†** Strengthen organs in pubic area: **LV-1†**
Treatment according to symptom:	Enuresis with dreams: **HT-7** Anorexia: **BL-20, ST-36**

Seminal Emission

Nocturnal Emission

Symptoms:	"Morning after" dizziness, palpitation, listlessness, lassitude, scant, yellow urine
Pulse:	Thready, rapid *Tongue:* Red body
Treatment:	Reduce heart fire: **HT-7, BL-15** Supplement kidney qi: **KI-3, BL-52**

Involuntary Emission (Spermatorrhea)

Symptoms:	Frequent emission, pallor, listlessness
Pulse:	Deep, feeble, thready, forceless *Tongue:* Pale body
Treatment:	Strengthen kidney function to control emission: **BL-23, KI-12, SP-6** Strengthen original qi by supplementing the conception vessel: **CV-4†, CV-6†**

Impotence

Kidney Yang Depletion

Symptoms:	Pallor, dizziness, blurring of vision, listlessness, soreness and weakness of lumbar region and knee, cold extremities, frequent urination
Pulse:	Deep, thready *Tongue:* Pale body, white coating
Treatment:	Supplement original qi: **CV-4†** Strengthen kidney yang: **GV-4†, BL-23†, KI-3** Raise yang qi to support kidney: **GV-20†**

Cardiosplenic Damage

Symptoms:	Palpitation and insomnia
Treatment:	Supplement heart and spleen: **BL-15, HT-7, SP-6**

Downpouring of Damp-Heat

Symptoms:	Bitter taste in mouth, thirst, dark red and hot urine, soreness and weakness in lower extremities
Pulse:	Soft, rapid *Tongue:* Sticky, yellow coating
Treatment:	Regulate spleen to drain damp and heat: **CV-3, SP-6, SP-9** Supplement stomach qi to reinforce spleen: **ST-36**

10 Selected Cardiovascular & Neurovascular Disorders

Bi (Obturation) Patterns

Wandering (Wind-Damp) Bi

Symptoms:	Moving pains in joints of extremities (wrists, elbows, knees, ankles) with limitation of movement, chills and fever
Pulse:	Floating and moderate
Tongue:	Thin, sticky coating
Treatment:	**BL-17, SP-10**, plus points according to areas affected (see below)

Dolorous (Cold-Damp) Bi

Symptoms:	Stabbing arthralgia that responds to warmth and is aggravated by cold; fixed location without local inflammation
Pulse:	Deep, tense, wiry
Tongue:	Thin, white coating
Treatment:	**BL-23, GV-4**, plus needling and moxibustion of points according to areas affected (see below)

Leaden (Damp) Bi

Symptoms:	Numbness of skin and muscles, heavy sensation of body and extremities, arthralgia with fixed pain, attacks provoked or aggravated by cloudy or damp weather
Pulse:	Deep, slow, soft
Tongue:	White, sticky coating
Treatment:	**ST-36, SP-5**, plus needling and moxibustion of points according to areas affected (see below)

(Continued)

Bi (Obturation) Patterns
(Continued)

Febrile Bi	
Symptoms:	Arthralgia with local inflammation, swelling, and tenderness; one or several joints possibly involved; possibly accompanied by fever and thirst
Pulse:	Rolling, rapid
Tongue:	Yellow coating
Treatment:	**GV-14, LI-11** plus needling using draining techniques according to areas affected (see below)
Treatment according to affected area:	Shoulder joint: **LI-15, TB-14, SI-9, SI-10** Scapula: **SI-11, SI-12, SI-14, BL-43** Elbow: **LI-11, LU-5, TB-10, TB-5, LI-4** Wrist: **TB-4, LI-5, SI-5, TB-5** Painful or numb fingers: **SI-3, LI-3, M-UE-22** (*baxie*) Stiff fingers: **SI-5, LI-4, SI-3** Hip joint: **GB-30, GB-29, BL-37, GB-39** Thigh: **BL-54, BL-36, GB-34** Knee: **ST-34, ST-35, M-LE-27** (*heding*), **M-LE-16** (*neixiyan*), **GB-34, GB-33, SP-9** Calf: **BL-57, BL-58** Ankle: **ST-41, SP-5, GB-40, BL-60, KI-3** Toes: **SP-4, BL-65, M-LE-8** (*bafeng*) Lumbar region: **GV-26, GV-12, GV-3** General aching: **SI-3, BL-62, SP-21, BL-17, GB-39**
Treatment according to symptoms:	Fever: **GV-14** Joint deformity: **BL-11**

Wei (Atony) Patterns

General:	Muscular flaccidity or atrophy of extremities with motor impairment
Points on affected area:	Upper limb: **LI-4, TB-5, LI-11, LI-14** Lower limb: **ST-31, ST-36, ST-41, GB-34, GB-39**

Lung Heat

Symptoms:	Occurs during or after febrile disease, accompanied by fever, cough, irritability, thirst, scant dark urine
Pulse:	Thready (or rolling) and rapid *Tongue:* Red with yellow fur
Treatment:	Dissipate lung heat: **LU-5, BL-13**

Damp-Heat

Symptoms:	Flaccid or swollen legs that are slightly hot to the touch, or hot sensation in soles of feet; fullness in chest and epigastrium, painful urination, hot or dark urine, sallow complexion, listlessness
Pulse:	Soft and rapid, or forceful and rapid *Tongue:* Yellow, sticky coating
Treatment:	Transform dampness to eliminate heat: **BL-20, SP-9**

Hepatorenal Qi and Essence Depletion

Symptoms:	Soreness and weakness of lumbar region, seminal emission, prospermia, leukorrhea, dizziness, blurring of vision
Pulse:	Thready, rapid *Tongue:* Red body
Treatment:	Supplement liver and kidney: **BL-18, BL-23**

Spinal Trauma

Symptoms:	History of trauma with flaccid, paralytic limbs; possibly accompanied by urinary and fecal incontinence
Pulse:	Moderate or hesitant *Tongue:* Pink or dark purple body, white coating
Treatment:	**M-BW-35** (*huatuo jiaji*) points at level of spinal injury Urinary incontinence: **CV-3, SP-6** Fecal incontinence: **BL-25, BL-32**

Note: Begin by needling the healthy side first, and then needle the affected side. Only yang channels are used in the treatment of *wei* patterns.

High Blood Pressure	
General Treatment:	Main points: **LI-11, ST-36, GB-20** Secondary points: **LI-4, PC-6, LV-3, ST-9** *Note:* In cases of extremely high blood pressure, avoid strong stimulation
Local Treatment:	Palpate and needle sensitive points: Head: **GV-20, BL-7** Neck: **GV-16, BL-10** Back: **BL-11, BL-12, BL-15** Upper limb: **LI-11, LI-10, PC-4, LI-4** Lower limb: **ST-36, GB-34** Chest and abdomen: **CV-17, CV-14**

Effulgent Liver Fire Type

Symptoms:	Dry mouth, constipation
Pulse:	Wiry, forceful
Tongue:	Yellow fur
Treatment:	Calm liver fire: Drain **LV-2, BL-18** Nourish spleen and lung to quell liver: Supplement **SP-3, LU-9**

Liver and Kidney Yin Depletion Type

Symptoms:	Dizziness, tinnitus, palpitations, insomnia
Pulse:	Wiry, fine, rapid
Tongue:	Red body
Treatment:	Nourish liver and kidney yin: Supplement **LV-3, LV-14, KI-3, KI-10**

(Continued)

High Blood Pressure
(Continued)

Extreme Damp Phlegm Type

Symptoms:	Thoracic oppression, upflow and nausea, heart palpitations, numb extremities
Pulse:	Wiry, slippery
Tongue:	Greasy
Treatment:	Clear phlegm from chest: **PC-5, PC-6, CV-17** Dry damp and transform phlegm: **SP-2, SP-3, ST-40, BL-20**

Mutual Depletion of Yin and Yang Type

Symptoms:	Heart palpitations, rapid breathing, dispiritedness, aching weakness of lumbar area and lower extremities, increased urination at night
Pulse:	Sunken, fine
Tongue:	Pale, red body
Treatment:	Nourish heart and kidney: **HT-7, HT-3, KI-3, KI-10** Fortify original yin and yang in lower burner: **CV-4†, GV-4†**

Internal Stirring of Liver Yang Type

Symptoms:	Severe headache, dizziness and confusion, convulsive spasm, fright inversion (sudden syncope)
Pulse:	Wiry, rapid
Tongue	Red body, thin yellow coat
Treatment:	Calm liver yang: Drain **BL-18, GB-20** Nourish liver yin: Supplement **LV-3, LV-8, LV-14**

11 Selected Obstetric and Gynecologic Disorders

Uterine Hemorrhage	
General Treatment:	Regulate penetrating and conception vessels: **CV-3** Empirical point for uterine bleeding: **SP-1** (moxa only)
Blood Heat Type	
Symptoms:	Sudden onset, bright red blood with foul odor; irritability, restlessness, insomnia, dizziness
Pulse:	Rapid
Tongue:	Red body with yellow coating
Treatment:	Regulate Conception and Penetrating Vessels: **CV-3** Regulate liver qi: **LV-8** Cool blood heat: **SP-10**
Supplementary Treatment:	Heat due to external pathogen: **LI-11** Heart fire repletion: **HT-8, PC-8** Liver fire repletion: **LV-3**
Qi Depletion	
Symptoms:	Continuous, scant bleeding, pinkish, dull blood, cold lower abdomen, chilliness, lassitude, anorexia, shortness of breath, apathy, pallor of face and lips
Pulse:	Thready, weak
Tongue:	Pale body
Treatment:	Raise yang qi: **CV-4†, GV-20†** Supplement spleen to control blood: **ST-36, SP-1†, SP-6** Supplement qi depletion in middle burner: **TB-4**

Uterine Prolapse

Qi Depletion

Symptoms:	Uterine prolapse with sinking sensation in the lower abdomen, lassitude, palpitations, shortness of breath, frequent urination, leukorrhagia
Pulse:	Weak *Tongue:* Pale body with thin coating
Treatment:	Supplement and raise qi: **CV-6†, GV-20†** Supplement middle burner qi: **CV-12†, ST-36†** Lift the uterus: **ST-29†**

Kidney Depletion

Symptoms:	Uterine prolapse with soreness and weakness in lower back and legs, bearing sensation in lower abdomen, dryness in vagina, frequent urination, dizziness, tinnitus
Pulse:	Deep, weak *Tongue:* Pink body
Treatment:	Supplement origin qi: **CV-4†** Supplement kidney and nourish tendons: **KI-6, LV-8** Lift the uterus: **M-CA-18** (*zigong*)

Metrorrhagia

General Symptoms:	Uterine bleeding at irregular cycles, accompanied by dizziness, heart palpitations, drained white complexion, cold extremities, perspiration, dull white fingernails and lips.
Pulse:	Deep, fine *Tongue:* Pale body
Treatment:	General points to control bleeding: **SP-1, SP-10**

Profuse metrorrhagia

Treatment	Secure qi to regulate the penetrating and conception Vessels: **CV-4, CV-6, CV-3** Stop bleeding and calm the liver: **SP-6, SP-2, SP-1**

Scant metrorrhagia

Treatment	Secure the lower origin: **CV-4, BL-23** Supplement spleen and kidney to conduct blood back to the channels: **BL-20†, SP-6†, LV-3†**

Irregular Menstruation
Early Menstruation

Blood Heat

Symptoms:	Short cycle, dark red, thick, copious flow, restlessness, fullness in chest, brown urine
Pulse:	Rapid, forceful *Tongue:* Red body with yellow coating
Treatment:	Cool blood heat: **LI-11, SP-10** Regulate and cool lower burner: **CV-3** Strengthen kidney yin to regulate menses: **KI-5** Cool liver fire: **LV-2** Cool yin depletion fire effulgence: **KI-2**

Qi Depletion

Symptoms:	Short cycle, profuse, thin, light red flow, lassitude, palpitation, shortness of breath, empty and heavy sensation in lower abdomen
Pulse:	Weak *Tongue:* Pale body
Treatment:	Reinforce qi: **CV-6†** Supplement blood: **CV-12, ST-36, SP-6**

Late Menstruation

Blood Depletion

Symptoms:	Scant, light red flow, empty and painful feeling in lower abdomen, emaciation, sallow complexion, lusterless skin, dizziness and blurred vision, palpitations, insomnia
Pulse:	Wcak, thready *Tongue:* Pink body with little or no coating
Treatment:	Regulate conception and penetrating vessels: **CV-4, CV-6** Strengthen lower yin channels: **SP-6** Clear dizziness and vision: **GV-20** Calm palpitations and insomnia: **HT-7**

Blood Cold

Symptoms:	Scant, dark flow, colic pain in lower abdomen that is slightly alleviated by warmth, cold limbs
Pulse:	Deep, slow *Tongue:* Thin, white coating
Treatment:	Warm uterus: **CV-3†, CV-4†, ST-29†** Supplement lower yin channels: **SP-6†**

(Continued)

Late Menstruation (Continued)	
Qi Stagnation	
Symptoms:	Scant, dark flow, distention and pain in lower abdomen, mental depression, congestion in chest relieved by belching, distention in hypochondrium and breasts
Pulse:	Wiry *Tongue:* Thin, white coating
Treatment:	Clear local stagnation: **ST-25, KI-13** Regulate spleen qi: **SP-8** Regulate liver qi: **LV-3** Relieve fullness in chest: **PC-6** Relieve distention in hypochondrium and breasts: **LV-14**

Irregular Cycles	
Liver Qi Stagnation	
Symptoms:	Irregular duration and quantity of flow, thick, sticky, purple flow, difficult flow, distention in hypochondrium and breast, distention and pain in lower abdomen, mental depression, frequent sighing
Pulse:	Wiry *Tongue:* Thin, white coating
Treatment:	Promote qi and blood in Conception and Penetrating Vessels: **CV-6, KI-14** Clear stagnated liver qi: **PC-5, LV-5** Relieve distention in hypochondrium and breasts: **CV-17, LV-14** Calm spirit and relieve depression: **HT-7, LV-3**
Kidney Depletion	
Symptoms:	Scant, light red flow, dizziness and tinnitus, weakness and aching in lumbar region and knees, frequent nocturnal urination, loose stools
Pulse:	Deep, weak *Tongue:* Pale body with thin coating
Treatment:	Supplement kidney qi and essence: **BL-23, CV-4, KI-8** Strengthen bones to relieve lumbar and knee pain: **M-BW-24** (*yaoyan*), **KI-10** Nourish marrow to relieve dizziness and tinnitus: **KI-3, GV-20**

Amenorrhea

Blood Conglomeration Type

General Symptoms:	Somber complexion, dry skin, weariness, lumbar pain, lower abdominal distention and hardness upon palpation, subtle, hidden pain; or lumbar and buttock pain extending to the back and shoulders; slightly disfluent urination, dry stools.
Pulse:	Deep, wiry *Tongue:* Red or purple body, petechiae or borders
Treatment:	Promote circulation in three foot-yin channels: **CV-3** Remove uterine stasis: **ST-29, BL-32** Activate and harmonize qi and blood: **LI-4, SP-6** Calm liver qi: **LV-2, LV-3** Activate blood to promote menstrual flow: **SP-20**

Blood Depletion Type

Symptoms:	Gradually decreasing appetite, slight fever, muscular wasting; somber yellow complexion, slightly puffy skin; worry and depression; counterflow cough, thoracic oppression, insomnia. Twisting pain in the abdomen
Pulse:	Slow, weak *Tongue:* Pale body with white coat
Treatment:	Fortify digestion, supplement construction & blood: **BL-18, BL-20†, BL-21†** Regulate construction and defense: **SP-10, CV-6** Abate agitation heat, resolve depression and binding: **SP-6** (For counterflow cough) clear heat and disinhibit qi in lung: **LU-9, LU-5** (If caused by parasite accumulation): **ST-4, ST-36**

Blood Dessication Type

Symptoms:	Complexion and lips somber white with a yellow tinge, generally haggard appearance, dry skin, dizziness and visual dazzling, weariness with desire for sleep, heart palpitations, rapid breathing, decreased food intake with poor digestion; dry bound stool, short scant urination; malar flush
Pulse:	Thready, wiry *Tongue:* Pale body with little coat
Treatment:	Promote flow of yang qi of entire body: **GV-14** Relieve taxation: **BL-43†** Nourish the kidneys and reinforce yin: **KI-7, BL-23** Regulate spleen, stomach, and center qi: **CV-12, BL-20, BL-21** Nourish the sea of blood: **SP-10†** Fortify the sea of qi: **CV-6†** Empirical point for all menstrual problems: moxa **M-BW-25**

Dysmenorrhea

Repletion Patterns

Depression of Liver Qi

Symptoms:	Premenstrual cramping pain, retarded, scant, dark purple menses with clots, distending pain in lower abdomen, distention in breasts and hypochondrium
Pulse:	Deep, wiry
Tongue:	Purplish body with purple petechiae on edges
Treatment:	Regulate conception and penetrating vessels: **CV-3** Course stagnated liver qi: **LI-4, LV-3** Relieve lower abdominal pain and distention: **KI-14, ST-28** Empirical point for dysmenorrhea: **BL-32**

Cold and Damp Stagnation in the Uterus

Symptoms:	Impeded, scant menses with clots and pain in lower abdomen, pain and cold in lower abdomen referring to waist and back, alleviated by warmth
Pulse:	Deep, wiry
Tongue:	Sticky, white coating
Treatment:	Regulate conception and penetrating vessels: **CV-3**† Invigorate blood flow and stop pain: **SP-8, SP-10** Warm channels and relieve local stasis: **ST-27**†, **ST-29**†

Depletion Patterns

Symptoms:	Lower abdominal pain at late stage of menstruation or post-menstrual pain is mild but persistent and alleviated by warmth or pressure. Menstrual flow is scant, pinkish. Possibly accompanied by chilliness, palpitation, dizziness.
Pulse:	Thready, forceless *Tongue:* Pale body, thin white fur
Treatment:	Warm and strengthen source qi: **CV-4**† Regulate spleen and kidney: **BL-20**†, **BL-23**† Strengthen spleen and stomach to promote blood formation: **ST-36, SP-6**

Leukorrhea

Spleen Depletion

Symptoms:	Profuse thick, white or light yellow discharge, pale or sallow complexion, lassitude, anorexia, loose stools, edema in lower limbs
Pulse:	Slow, weak *Tongue:* Pale body
Treatment:	Stabilize girdling vessel: **GB-26** Regulate conception and girdling vessels: **CV-6** Check discharge: **BL-30** Reinforce spleen to transform damp: **ST-36, SP-9**

Kidney Depletion

Symptoms:	Profuse, continuous, thin, transparent or white discharge, soreness in lower back, cold sensation in lower abdomen, frequent and profuse urination, loose stools
Pulse:	Deep *Tongue:* Pale body with thin coating
Treatment:	Reinforce yang qi and supplement kidney: **CV-4†, BL-23†, KI-7** Stabilize conception and girdling vessels: **KI-12, GB-26**

Damp-Heat

Symptoms:	Profuse, sticky, viscous, foul-smelling yellow discharge, vulvar itching, dry stool, scant yellow urine
Pulse:	Soft, rapid *Tongue:* Sticky, yellow coating
Treatment:	Clear damp-heat in lower warmer: **CV-3** Check discharge: **BL-32** Supplement spleen to transform damp and reduce liver fire: **SP-6** Relieve vulvar itching: **LV-5**

Blood Heat

Symptoms:	Reddish yellow discharge, bitter taste in mouth, dry throat, irritability with feverish sensation, palpitations, insomnia
Pulse:	Wiry, rapid *Tongue:* Yellow coating
Treatment:	Drain heat in lower yin channels: **SP-6** Cool blood heat: **SP-10** Resolve pathogenic heat: **LI-11**

Morning Sickness

Gastrosplenic Depletion	
Symptoms:	Nausea and vomiting of liquid or undigested food immediately after meals, fullness and distention in the chest, lassitude and somnolence
Pulse:	Slippery and weak (first trimester) *Tongue:* Pale body, white coating
Treatment:	Calm the center, stop nausea, promote downflow of stomach qi: **PC-6, CV-12, CV-13, ST-36, SP-4**

Liver Qi Invades Stomach	
Symptoms:	Vomiting of bitter or sour liquid, epigastric fullness, hypochondriac pain, frequent belching and sighing, mental depression, dizziness, pain or swelling in eyes.
Pulse:	Wiry (first trimester) *Tongue:* Yellowish coating
Treatment:	Regulate liver qi: **PC-6, LV-3** Downbear stomach qi counterflow: **CV-17, CV-12, ST-36**

Prolonged Labor

Qi and Blood Depletion	
Symptoms:	Dull, paroxysmal labor pains, mild heavy or distending sensation, or profuse, light colored hemorrhage; possibly pallor, lassitude, palpitation, shortness of breath
Pulse:	Weak *Tongue:* Pale body
Treatment:	Supplement qi and blood: **SP-6†, ST-36†** Promote delivery: **BL-67†**

Qi and Blood Stagnation	
Symptoms:	Sharp pains in waist and abdomen, scant, dark red hemorrhage, dark cyanotic complexion, mental depression, fullness in chest and epigastrium, frequent nausea.
Pulse:	Deep, forceful *Tongue:* Dark body
Treatment:	Regulate qi and blood to clear stagnation: **LI-4, SP-6** Promote delivery: **BL-67†**

Malposition of Fetus	
Treatment:	Empirical point for turning a malpositioned fetus: **BL-67** (continuous indirect moxibustion for fifteen to twenty minutes, several times daily).

Insufficient Lactation

General Treatment:	Empirical point for promoting lactation: **SI-1** Activate upper burner qi: **CV-17** Local point to stimulate lactation: **ST-18**

Qi and Blood Depletion

Symptoms:	Insufficiency or absence of lactation after delivery, no pain in breasts, pallor, dry skin, palpitations, lassitude, anorexia, loose stools
Pulse:	Weak, thready *Tongue:* Pale body with little coating
Treatment:	Supplement stomach and spleen to promote blood and milk formation: **BL-20, ST-36, SP-6**

Liver Qi Stagnation

Symptoms:	Retention of milk after delivery, distending pain in breasts, fullness in chest, pain in hypochondrium, distention in epigastrium, anorexia
Pulse:	Wiry *Tongue:* Pink body
Treatment:	Relieve liver qi stagnation: **LV-3, LV-14** Regulate qi in chest and restore milk flow: **PC-6**

Acute Mastitis

General Symptoms:	Redness, swelling, heat, and pain in breast; possibly accompanied by chills, fever, nausea, irritability, thirst
Pulse:	Wiry, rapid *Tongue:* Red body, thin yellow coat
Treatment:	Calm liver: **LV-3** Ease pain and distention in breast: **GB-41** Relieve pressure in chest: **CV-17** Promote local qi circulation: **GB-21, ST-18** Reduce chills and fever: **LI-4, TB-5** Local point for reducing breast pain and promoting lactation: **ST-16** (oblique puncture)

12   Selected Pediatric Disorders

Infantile Convulsion	
Acute	
Symptoms:	High fever, coma, upward-staring eyes, clenched jaws, rattle in throat, tetanic contraction, opisthotonos, cyanosis
Pulse:	Rapid, wiry
Treatment:	Eliminate intense heat: **M-UE-1** *to* **-5** (*shixuan*) (bleed) Promote relaxation and relieve spasm: **M-HN-3** (*yintang*) Resuscitation point: **GV-26** Calm liver wind: **LV-3**
Treatment according to symptom:	Coma: emergency points to clear heat: **PC-8, KI-1** Protracted convulsions: calm liver and gallbladder to relax the tendons: **LV-2, GB-34** Regulate taiyang and Governing Vessel to clear the mind: **SI-3, BL-60** Continuous high fever: drain heat pathogen in yang channels: **GV-14, LI-4, LI-11**
Chronic	
Symptoms:	Emaciation, pallor, lassitude, lethargy, half-closed eyes, intermittent convulsion, cold extremities, loose stools with undigested food, profuse clear urine
Pulse:	Deep, weak
Treatment:	Reinforce Conception and Governing Vessels: **CV-4†, GV-20, GV-24** Reinforce qi and blood: **SP-6, ST-36** Supplement spleen and kidney yang depletion: **CV-12†, BL-20†, BL-23†** Nourish yin and blood: **KI-2, LV-3**

Infantile Diarrhea

General Symptoms:	Abdominal distention, borborygmi, intermittent abdominal pain relieved after defecation; stools with strong, fetid odor and possibly interspersed with milk curd; eructation, anorexia
Pulse:	Rolling, full, or rolling, rapid *Tongue:* Yellow, sticky coating
Treatment:	Relieve food stagnation in stomach: **CV-6, CV-11** Adjust function of large intestine: **ST-25, ST-37** Empirical point for infantile diarrhea: **M-UE-9** (*sifeng*) (bleed) If due to exogenous cold add: **LI-4** If due to damp-heat add: **LI-11, SP-9**

Infantile Malnutrition

General Symptoms:	Gradual onset of slight fevers or tidal fevers in afternoon, dryness in mouth, abdominal distention, diarrhea with foul odor, cloudy urine, anorexia, and irritable crying; progresses to abdominal distention with protruding umbilicus, sallow complexion, emaciation, scaly or dry skin
Pulse:	Weak *Tongue:* Unclean-looking, sticky, or no coating
Treatment:	Harmonize stomach and clear heat: **ST-10** Supplement earth and replenish qi: **SP-3, ST-36** Invigorate yang qi of spleen and kidney: **BL-20†, BL-23†** Empirical point for infantile malnutrition: **M-UE-9** (*sifeng*) (bleed) If due to parasites: **M-LE-34** (*baichongwo*)

Parotitis (Mumps)

General Symptoms:	Unilateral or bilateral swelling of parotid region, accompanied by thirst, constipation, deep yellow urine
Pulse:	Floating, rapid *Tongue:* Yellow, sticky coating
Treatment:	Dispel heat in triple burner channel: **TB-5** Dispel heat in hand yangming channel: **LI-4, LI-11** Disperse obstruction in local channels: **ST-6, TB-17**

13 Selected Dermatological Disorders

Urticaria	
General Symptoms:	Abrupt onset of raised, itching wheals of various size; may occur intermittently and repeatedly over long periods of time
General Treatment:	Eliminate heat from skin and muscles: **LI-4, LI-11** Cool heat in blood: **SP-10, BL-40**
Wind-Heat	
Symptoms:	Red rashes with severe itching
Pulse:	Floating, rapid
Tongue	Red body, thin yellow coating
Treatment:	Cool heat in yang channels: **GV-14**
Wind-damp type	
Symptoms:	White or light red rashes accompanied by heavy sensation in body
Pulse:	Floating, slow
Tongue:	White, sticky coating
Treatment:	Drain dampness: **SP-6, SP-9**
Gastrointestinal Heat Bind	
Symptoms:	Red rashes with abdominal or epigastric pain, constipation, or diarrhea
Pulse:	Rapid
Tongue:	Thin, yellow coating
Treatment:	Drain heat in stomach and intestines: **ST-25, ST-36**

Erysipelas	
General Symptoms:	Sudden appearance of red patches diffusely spread over the skin, clearly demarcated and with burning pain.
General Treatment:	Eliminate heat in yangming: **LI-4, LI-11** Eliminate blood heat: **PC-3** (bleed), **SP-10** Eliminate damp-heat: **BL-40** (bleed)
Wind-Heat	
Symptoms:	Urticaria accompanied by chills, fever, acute headache
Pulse:	Floating, rapid
Tongue:	Red body with thin, yellow coating
Treatment:	Clear channel heat: **GV-14** Dispel wind: **GB-20**
Damp-Heat	
Symptoms:	Urticaria accompanied by fever, irritability, thirst, oppression in chest, anorexia, constipation, dark urine
Pulse:	Soft, rapid
Tongue:	Yellow, sticky coating
Treatment:	Clear heat from channels: **GV-14** Drain dampness: **ST-36, SP-9** Relieve constipation: **TB-6**
Pathogenic Invasion Into Interior	
Symptoms:	Urticaria accompanied by high fever, vomiting, delirium, convulsion
Treatment:	Drain interior heat: **PC-8** Reduce high fever: bleed twelve *jing*-well points of hands

Herpes Zoster	
General Symptoms:	Small bead-like vesicles forming a belt-like pattern in lumbar and hypochondriac regions, with severe burning pain, inflammation, and hot skin
Treatment:	Eliminate heat in yangming: **LI-4, LI-11** Eliminate blood heat: **SP-10, BL-40** (bleed) Eliminate damp-heat: **LV-3, GB-34** Treat local area: local **M-BW-35** (*huatuo jiaji*)

Furuncle and Lymphangitis	
General Symptoms:	A hard, yellow or purple blister, usually accompanied by chills and fever. Usually occurs on head, face, or extremities.
Treatment:	Empirical point for furuncle: **GV-10** Regulate qi of yang channels: **GV-12** Cool the blood: **PC-4** Resolve exterior pathogens: **LI-4** Clear blood heat and toxins: **BL-40** (bleed)

14 Selected Eye, Ear, Nose, and Throat Disorders

Deafness and Tinnitus	
General Treatment:	Tinnitus: regulate qi of liver and gallbladder channels: **LV-2, GB-41** Sudden deafness: empirical point for sudden deafness: **TB-16** Local and distal points selected from channels passing through the ear: **TB-17, TB-21, GB-2, TB-2, GB-43, TB-3**

Repletion type	
Symptoms:	Continuous ringing of the ear, unrelieved by pressure; sudden deafness.

Liver-Gallbladder Fire Effulgence	
Symptoms:	Flushed face, dry mouth, irritability, bitter taste in mouth, hypochondriac pain
Pulse:	Wiry *Tongue:* Red body, yellow coat
Treatment:	Cool liver-gallbladder fire: **LV-2, GB-41**

Pathogenic Wind Invasion	
Symptoms:	Headache, heavy sensation in head, nasal obstruction
Pulse:	Floating and rapid *Tongue:* Red body, thin coating
Treatment:	Resolve exterior to dispel wind pathogen: **LI-4, TB-5**

Depletion Type	
Symptoms:	Intermittent ringing of ear, aggravated by stress and strain, somewhat alleviated by pressure; gradually intensifying deafness. Accompanying symptoms include dizziness, blurring of vision, low back pain, lassitude
Pulse:	Thready, weak *Tongue:* Pale body, thin, white coating
Treatment:	Supplement kidney qi: **BL-23†, GV-4†, KI-3** Nourish liver yin to reduce depletion fire: **LV-3** Supplement yin and blood: **SP-6**

Epistaxis (Nosebleed)	
General Treatment:	Local and distal points on channels passing through the nose: **LI-4, LI-20, GV-23**

Heat Repletion in Lung and Stomach	
Symptoms:	Nosebleed accompanied by fever, cough, thirst, foul breath, constipation
Pulse:	Forceful, rapid *Tongue:* Red body with yellow coating
Treatment:	Reduce lung and stomach heat: **LU-11, ST-44**

Yin Depletion Fire Effulgence	
Symptoms:	Nosebleed accompanied by malar flush, dry mouth, "fever in five hearts" (palms, soles, and chest), afternoon fever, night sweating
Pulse:	Thready, rapid *Tongue:* Dry, yellow coating
Treatment:	Supplement kidney yin to reduce fire: **KI-6**

Congestion, Swelling, and Pain in the Eye	
Symptoms:	Congestion, swelling, pain and burning sensation of the eye, photophobia, lacrimation, sticky discharge

Invasion of Exogenous Wind Heat	
Symptoms:	Headache, fever
Pulse:	Floating, rapid
Treatment:	Disperse wind-heat: **TB-5, GB-20** Dispel local heat and stagnation: **BL-1, M-HN-9** (*taiyang*) (bleed)

Upward Disturbance of Liver and Gallbladder Fire	
Symptoms:	Bitter taste in mouth, irritability with feverish sensation, constipation
Pulse:	Wiry *Tongue:* White coating
Treatment:	Reduce liver and gallbladder fire: **LV-2, LV-3, GB-37**

Rhinorrhea	
General Symptoms:	Nasal obstruction, loss of sense of smell, yellow fetid nasal discharge; possibly accompanied by cough, dull pain, cloudiness and heaviness of frontal region of head
Pulse:	Wiry, rapid *Tongue:* Red body, thin yellow coating
Treatment:	Activate lung yin: **LU-7** Reduce heat in large intestine channel: **LI-4, LI-20** Relieve nasal obstruction: **M-HN-3** (*yintang*) Dispel wind to relieve headache: **GB-20** Disperse heat to relieve headache: **M-HN-9** (*taiyang*)

Toothache	
Stomach Fire	
Symptoms:	Severe pain with foul breath, thirst, constipation
Pulse:	Forceful, rapid *Tongue:* Yellow coating
Treatment:	Drain pathogenic heat from yangming channel: **LI-4** (contralateral) Drain stomach fire: **ST-44** Clear stagnation from local area: **ST-6, ST-7**
Wind-Heat	
Symptoms:	Gingival swelling and pain, thirst with preference for cold beverages, chills and fever
Pulse:	Floating, rapid *Tongue:* Red body with yellow coating
Treatment:	Cool heat in shaoyang channel: **TB-2** Expel wind: **TB-5, GB-20** Cool heat and relieve stagnation in yangming channel: **LI-4, ST-6, ST-7**
Kidney Depletion	
Symptoms:	Intermittent dull pain, loose teeth, no foul breath
Pulse:	Thready, rapid *Tongue:* Red body
Treatment:	Nourish kidney yin: **KI-3** Relive local pain stagnation: **ST-6, ST-7**

Sore Throat	
Heat Repletion	
Symptoms:	Abrupt onset, with chills, fever, headache, congestion and soreness in throat, thirst, constipation
Pulse:	Floating, rapid
Tongue:	Red body with thin, yellow coating
Treatment:	Drain lung heat: **LU-11** (bleed) Resolve pathogens in exterior: **LI-4** Drain stomach channel heat: **ST-44** Relieve local stagnation pain: **SI-17**
Yin Depletion	
Symptoms:	Gradual onset, with little or no fever, intermittent sore throat pain, dryness in throat which becomes aggravated at night, heat sensation in palms and soles
Pulse:	Thready, rapid
Tongue:	Red body with no coating
Treatment:	Nourish kidney yin and drain lung fire: **KI-3, LU-10** Relieve local pain: **CV-23** Open conception and yin motility vessels to activate kidney and move fluids: **KI-6 LU-7** Relieve local pain: **LI-18**

Optic Atrophy

General Treatment:	Regulate qi in local area: **GB-20, BL-1, M-HN-8** (*qiuhou*), **GB-39**

Liver and Kidney Yin Depletion

Symptoms:	Dryness of eyes, blurred vision, dizziness, tinnitus, nocturnal emission, aching of lower back
Pulse:	Thready, weak
Tongue:	Red body with scant coating
Treatment:	Supplement liver and kidney yin: **LV-3, KI-3** Subdue liver and kidney yang: **BL-18, BL-23**

Blood and Qi Depletion

Symptoms:	Blurred vision, dyspnea, taciturnity, lassitude, anorexia, loose stools
Pulse:	Thready, weak
Tongue:	Pale body with thin, white coating
Treatment:	Supplement qi and blood: **SP-6, ST-36**

Liver Qi Stagnation

Symptoms:	Blurred vision, emotional depression, dizziness, vertigo, hypochondriac pain, bitter taste in mouth, dry throat
Pulse:	Wiry
Treatment:	Relieve liver qi stagnation: **LV-3, LV-14, GB-34**

15   Selected Endocrinological Disorders

<table>
<tr><td colspan="2" align="center">**Diabetes**
Wasting Thirst</td></tr>
<tr><td>*General Symptoms:*</td><td>Sweet-tasting urine, thirst with desire to drink, excessive urination, thinness despite high food intake, gradual emaciation, fatigue and lack of strength, genital itching and irritation; in later stages, purulent abscesses.</td></tr>
<tr><td colspan="2">**Upper Wasting**</td></tr>
<tr><td>*Symptoms:*</td><td>Parched throat, great thirst, desire for liquids, normal stool, clear or red, disfluent urine.</td></tr>
<tr><td>*Pulse:*</td><td>Flooding, rapid   *Tongue:* Fissured, red sides and tip, thin yellow fur</td></tr>
<tr><td>*Treatment:*</td><td>Clear upper burner lung heat: **BL-13, LU-11, LI-4**
Downbear counterflow to resolve heat: **ST-36, SP-6**
Supplement yin and moisten yang: **LV-2, KI-1**</td></tr>
<tr><td colspan="2">**Middle Wasting**</td></tr>
<tr><td>*Symptoms:*</td><td>Thirst, extreme hunger, consumption of food and drink in double quantities but retaining thin appearance, spontaneous persiration, rather copious urination, firm stools.</td></tr>
<tr><td>*Pulse:*</td><td>Slippery, forceful   *Tongue:* Yellow, dry fur</td></tr>
<tr><td>*Treatment:*</td><td>Clear stomach heat and regulate the middle burner: **LI-11, PC-6, ST-36, CV-12**</td></tr>
<tr><td colspan="2">**Lower Wasting**</td></tr>
<tr><td>*Symptoms:*</td><td>Irregular urination, sediment in urine, agitated thirst with desire to drink, sallow, drawn complexion, earlobes parched and blackened, turbid urine, with a bran-like or greasy froth</td></tr>
<tr><td>*Pulse:*</td><td>Deep, fine, rapid   *Tongue:* Red body</td></tr>
<tr><td>*Treatment:*</td><td>Supplement the kidneys and nourish yin: **CV-4, BL-23, LV-2, KI-6, KI-1**

Relieve thoracic oppression and regulate urinary excretion: **SP-6, PC-6**</td></tr>
</table>

16   Selected Respiratory Disorders

Common Cold	
Wind-cold	
Symptoms:	Chills, aversion to cold, mild fever, no perspiration, headache, nasal obstruction, rhinitis, aching joints; possibly itching throat, cough
Pulse:	Floating, tense
Tongue:	Thin, white coating
Treatment:	Eliminate wind, resolve the exterior: **GV-16, GB-20, BL-12** Relieve headache and nasal obstruction: **LU-7** Cause perspiration to resolve exterior: **LI-4, KI-7** Dispel wind in facial region: **M-HN-9** (*taiyang*)**, LI-20**
Wind-heat	
Symptoms:	Fever, aversion to wind, perspiration, distended sensation in head, thirst, hacking cough, dry, congested, sore throat.
Pulse:	Floating, rapid
Tongue:	Thin, yellow coating
Treatment:	Clear heat in yang channels: **GV-14** Expel wind and heat: **LI-4, TB-5, GB-20** Cool the throat: **LU-10, LU-11** (bleed)
Prophylaxis:	During "cold season," daily moxibustion at **BL-12** and **ST-36** will strengthen the body's defensive qi and prevent penetration of exogenous pathogens.

Asthma	
Depletion	
Lung Depletion Asthma	
Symptoms:	Short, quick breathing, difficulty on inhalation, weak and low voice, sweating on exertion, weak cough
Pulse:	Weak, depleted *Tongue:* Pale body
Treatment:	Reinforce lung qi: **BL-13**† Strengthen lung-metal by supplementing earth: **LU-9, SP-3, ST-36**
Kidney Depletion Asthma	
Symptoms:	Dyspnea upon exertion, severe wheezing, difficulty on exhalation, chilliness with cold extremities, general lassitude
Pulse:	Deep, thready, feeble *Tongue:* Pale body
Treatment:	Reinforce kidney qi: **BL-23**†, **GV-4**†, **CV-6**† Regulate respiratory qi: **CV-17**
Chronic Persistent Asthma	
Garlic moxibustion on **GV-12, BL-43** will strengthen the respiratory function. Direct or indirect moxa on **BL-20** and **CV-12** will strengthen splenic yang and prevent mucus production.	

Cough *Exogenous*	
Wind-Cold Cough	
Symptoms:	Headache, aversion to cold, chills and fever, nasal obstruction and discharge, thin white sputum, no perspiration
Pulse:	Floating
Tongue:	Thin, white coating
Treatment:	Eliminate wind and resolve exterior: **LU-7, LI-4**† Activate dispersing function of lung: **BL-13**† Moisten lung to relieve cough: **LU-5**
Wind-Heat Cough	
Symptoms:	Choking cough with yellow, thick sputum, headache, sore throat, aversion to wind, fever without chills, thirst, sweating
Pulse:	Floating, rapid
Tongue:	Thin, yellow coating
Treatment:	Eliminate wind and secure exterior: **GB-20, TB-5** Reduce fever: **LI-11, GV-14** Cool pain and swelling in throat: **LU-11** (bleed)

Cough
Endogenous

Cough from Lung Yin Depletion

Symptoms:	Dry cough, little or no sputum, dry or sore throat. Possibly bloody sputum, hemoptysis, afternoon fever, malar flush.
Pulse:	Feeble, rapid
Tongue:	Red body with thin coating
Treatment:	Regulate respiratory function: **BL-13, LU-1** Supplement yin, activate descending function of lung: **LU-7, KI-6** Stop hemoptysis: **LU-6, BL-17**

Cough from Spleen Yang Depletion

Symptoms:	Cough with excessive sputum, more severe in winter, anorexia, listlessness
Pulse:	Deep, slow, or rolling
Tongue:	Thick, sticky, slippery, white coating
Treatment:	Activate lung qi: **BL-13†** Supplement yang to dispel pathogen: **BL-12†, GV-14†** Eliminate wind and cold: **LU-7, LI-4†**

Phlegm-Heat Asthma

Symptoms:	Rapid, coarse breathing, oppression in chest, thick yellow sputum, fever, restlessness, dry mouth
Pulse:	Rapid, rolling, forceful
Tongue:	Thick, yellow coating
Treatment:	Resolve phlegm in chest: **PC-5 CV-22** Cool lung heat: **LU-5** Calm breathing: **M-BW-1b** (*dingchuan*)

Essentials of Chinese Acupuncture and *Chinese Acupuncture and Moxibustion* recommend **ST-40** instead of **PC-5**. Clinical experience, however, shows that the combination of **PC-5** with **CV-22** is far more effective for phlegm in the upper burner. **ST-40** (with **SP-3**) should be used for middle burner generated phlegm (i.e., splenic yang depletion phlegm).

17   Selected Emotional Disorders

Melancholia	
Binding Depression of Liver Qi	
Symptoms:	Mental depression, thoracic distress, hypochondriac pain, abdominal distention, belching, anorexia, abdominal pain, vomiting, irregular bowel movements
Pulse:	Wiry
Tongue	Thin, sticky coating
Treatment:	Regulate qi in upper burner: **CV-17** Soothe liver to relieve binding depression: **LV-3, BL-18** Harmonize stomach, promote descending function: **CV-12, ST-36** Strengthen spleen to help harmonize stomach: **SP-4**
Depressed Qi Transforms into Fire	
Symptoms:	Headache, dry mouth with bitter taste, irritability, thoracic distress, hypochondriac distention, acid regurgitation, constipation, reddening of eyes, tinnitus
Pulse:	Wiry, rapid
Tongue	Thin, sticky coating
Treatment:	Dispel liver and gallbladder fire: **LV-2, GB-43** Relieve thoracic and hypochondriac distress: **TB-6, GB-34** Harmonize upper orifice of stomach to relieve acid upflow: **CV-13**
Plum-stone Globus (Phlegm Stagnation in Throat)	
Symptoms:	Feeling of a lump in the throat
Pulse:	Wiry, rolling
Tongue:	Thin, sticky coating
Treatment:	Soothe liver: **LV-2** Relieve upper burner phlegm and precipitate throat qi: **PC-7, CV-22** Relieve depression in chest, regulate upper burner qi: **PC-6, CV-17** Transform phlegm in middle burner: **ST-40**

(Continued)

Melancholia
(Continued)

Blood Depletion

Symptoms:	Grief without cause, capricious joy or anger, suspiciousness, fearfulness, palpitations, irritability, insomnia, sudden thoracic distress, hiccough, sudden aphonia, convulsion, syncope
Pulse:	Wiry, thready
Tongue:	Thin, white coating
Treatment:	Soothe liver to release depression: **LV-3** Nourish blood and calm the spirit: **SP-6, BL-14, HT-7** Relieve thoracic depression: **PC-6, CV-17** Precipitate qi to check hiccough: **SP-4, CV-22** Relieve aphonia: **HT-5, CV-23** Stop convulsion by regulating qi flow and tendons: **LI-4, GB-34** Restore consciousness: **GV-26, KI-1**

Hysteria

Symptoms:	Melancholia, paraphrenia, suspiciousness, paraphobia, palpitation, irritability, somnolence, etc. Possibly suffocating sensation, hiccough, aphonia, convulsion. In severe cases: loss of consciousness and syncope.
Pulse:	Wiry, thready
General Treatment:	Calm the spirit, nourish yin-blood: **CV-14, HT-7, SP-6**
Treatment according to symptoms	Suffocating sensation: **PC-6, CV-17** Hiccough: **SP-4, CV-22** Aphonia: **HT-5, CV-23** Convulsion: **LI-4, LV-3** Loss of consciousness, syncope: **GV-26, KI-1**

Palpitation and Anxiety

General Treatment:	Regulate the heart: **BL-15, CV-14** Calm the spirit: **HT-7** Regulate the blood: **PC-6**

Mental Disturbance

Symptoms:	Palpitation, fear and fright, irritability, restlessness
Pulse:	Small, rapid *Tongue:* Pale, red body, thin white coating
Treatment:	Strengthen qi: **CV-6** Fortify blood production: **BL-20, BL-21, ST-36**

Stirring of Endogenous Phlegm-Fire

Symptoms:	Irritability, restlessness, dream-disturbed sleep
Pulse:	Rapid, rolling *Tongue:* Yellow coating
Treatment:	Transform phlegm: **ST-40** Downbear fire: **GB-34**

Yin Depletion Fire Effulgence

Symptoms:	Palpitation, restlessness, irritability, insomnia, dizziness, blurred vision, tinnitus
Pulse:	Thready, rapid *Tongue:* Red body with little coating
Treatment:	Supplement kidney: **KI-3, BL-23** Clear heart fire: **BL-14**

Retention of Harmful Fluid

Symptoms:	Expectoration of thick phlegm, fullness in the chest and epigastrium, lassitude
Pulse:	Wiry, rolling *Tongue:* White coating
Treatment:	Move fluid: **CV-9, SP-9, BL-22** Invigorate yang: **CV-4, CV-17** Strengthen spleen and stomach: **ST-36**

Manic-Depressive Disorders

General Treatment:	Restore mental clarity: **GV-26** Dispel heat: **LI-11** Stabilize spirit: **SP-1**

Depressive Disorders

Symptoms:	Gradual onset, depression and dejection, mental dullness, progressing to incoherent speech, mood swings, taciturnity, somnolence, anorexia
Pulse:	Thready and wiry, or rolling and wiry *Tongue:* Thin, sticky fur
Treatment:	Clear the heart: **BL-15** Remove liver stagnation: **BL-18** Promote spleen qi circulation: **BL-20** Fortify the spirit: **HT-7** Transform phlegm stagnation in middle burner: **ST-40**

Manic Disorders

Symptoms:	Sudden onset, irritability, insomnia, loss of appetite, progressing to excessive motor activity with increased energy and violent behavior
Pulse:	Wiry, rolling, and rapid *Tongue:* Sticky, yellow coating
Treatment:	Clear the mind: **GV-26** Reduce heat in governing channel: **GV-16, GV-14** Clear the heart and transform phlegm: **PC-6, ST-40**
Treatment according to symptoms:	Clear heat in pericardium channel: **PC-8, PC-7** Clear heat in governing and yangqiao channels: **GV-23, GV-16, BL-62** Clear heat in yangming channels: **LI-11, ST-6** Manic cases with extreme heat: bleed 12 *jing*-well points on hands
Classical Treatment:	Sun Simo's "Thirteen Ghost Points" (bleed in succession): **GV-26, LU-11, SP-1, PC-7, BL-62, GV-16, ST-6, CV-24, PC-8, GV-23, CV-1, LI-11, M-HN-37** (*haiquan,* also called *shexiazhongfeng*) From the *Zhenjiu Dacheng:* First, restore stability to the center by needling **ST-36**. Then, needle Alarm-*mu* points of organs corresponding to the disturbed emotions according to five phase theory. One source says needle *all* the alarm points of the yin organs.

Epilepsy	
During Seizure	
Symptoms:	**Note:** *Though not strictly an emotional disorder, epilepsy has been included here because of its association with brain function disturbances, as well as due to its association in traditional Chinese medicine with the Spirit.*
	Preceded by dizziness, headache, oppression in chest, progressing to collapse with loss of consciousness, pallor, clenched jaws, upward staring eyes, convulsions, foaming at the mouth, incoherent raving, urinary and fecal incontinence
Pulse:	Wiry, rolling
Tongue:	Sticky, white coating
Treatment:	Resuscitation points: **GV-26, CV-15**
	Calm heart: **PC-5**
	Transform phlegm: **ST-40**
	Dispel wind: **LV-3**
After Seizure	
Symptoms:	Listlessness, lusterless complexion, dizziness, palpitations, anorexia, phlegm stagnation: **CV-12, ST-40**
	Severe qi and blood depletion: **CV-4†, ST-36†**

18   Selected Neurological Disorders

Facial Paralysis	
Symptoms:	Sudden onset, incomplete closing of eye, tearing, drooping of angle of mouth, salivation, inability to frown or raise eyebrow, blow out the cheek, show the teeth, or whistle. Possibly accompanied by pain in mastoid region or headache
Pulse:	Floating and tense, or floating and slow
Tongue:	Thin, white coating
General Treatment:	Clear the channels: **LI-4, LV-3** Eliminate wind from involved channels: use **LI-4** as distal point, add local points according to palpation: **TB-17, GB-14, M-HN-9** (*taiyang*), **SI-18, ST-7, ST-4, ST-6**
Treatment according to symptom:	Headache: **GB-20** Profuse sputum: **ST-40** Difficulty in frowning or raising eye: **BL-2, TB-23** Difficulty in sniffing: **LI-20** Incomplete closing of eye: **BL-2, BL-1, GB-1, M-HN-6** *(yuyao)*, **TB-23** Deviation of philtrum: **GV-26** Inability to show teeth: **ST-3** Tinnitus and deafness: **GB-2** Twitching of eyelid and mouth: **LV-3** Tenderness at mastoid region: **TB-5, GB-12**

Windstrike	
Severe Type (Zang-Fu Organs Attacked)	
Tense Syndrome	
Symptoms:	Eyes staring, clenched jaws, clenched fists, anhidrosis, retention of urine, constipation
Pulse:	Wiry, rolling, forceful *Tongue:* Yellow, sticky coating
General Treatment:	Raise yang in governing vessel: **GV-26, GV-20** Drain heat in upper body: 12 *jing*-well points of hands (bleed) Conduct upper body heat downward: **KI-1**
Symptomatic Treatment:	Clenched jaws: local: **ST-6, ST-7**; distal: **LI-4** Gurgling with sputum: **CV-22, PC-5, ST-40** Aphasia with stiff tongue: local: **GV-15, CV-23**; distal: **HT-5**
Flaccid syndrome	
Symptoms:	Eyes closed, mouth agape, relaxed hands, hidrosis, incontinence of urine and feces, cold limbs
Pulse:	Feeble *Tongue:* Limp
Treatment:	Revive yang and avert collapse: **CV-4, CV-6, CV-8†** (on salt)
Mild Type (Channels and Connecting Vessels Attacked)	
General Symptoms:	Hemiplegia, motor impairment, dizziness, aphasia
Pulse:	Floating, slippery *Tongue:* White sticky coating

General Treatment:	Eliminate wind pathogen
	    in the upper body: **GV-20, GV-16, BL-7**
	    in the upper extremities: **LI-4, TB-5, LI-11, LI-15**
	    in the lower extremities: **GB-30, GB-34, ST-36, ST-41**
	    in the face (mouth awry): **ST-4, ST-6**

Prophylaxis:	Frequent moxibustion on **ST-36** and **GB-39**
Ascendant hyperactivity of liver yang:	Reduce wind and calm the liver: **GB-20, LV-3** Supplement kidney yin to nourish the liver: **KI-3, SP-6**
Fire effulgence in the heart and liver	Cool fire in heart and liver: **PC-7, LV-2** Supplement yin to cool fire: **KI-3**

Headache
Repletion Pattern

Wind Pathogen Invades the Channels

Symptoms:	Violent, boring pain that may extend to nape and back
Pulse:	Wiry
Tongue:	Thin, white coating
Symptomatic Treatment:	Occipital (taiyang channels affected): **SI-3, GB-20, BL-60** Frontal (yangming channels affected): **LI-4, ST-8, M-HN-3** (*yintang*), **GV-23, ST-44** Temporal (shaoyang channels affected): **TB-5, GB-8, M-HN-9** (*taiyang*), **GB-41** Parietal (jueyin and taiyang channels affected): **SI-3, GV-20, LV-3, BL-67**

Ascendant Hyperactivity of Liver Yang

Symptoms:	Headache with blurred vision, severe temporal pain, irritability, flushed face, bitter taste in mouth
Pulse:	Wiry, rapid
Tongue:	Red body with yellow coating
Treatment:	Reduce liver wind in head: **GB-20, GV-20, GB-5** Calm liver yang and reduce channel heat: **LV-2, GB-43**

Depletion Pattern

Qi and Blood Depletion

Symptoms:	Persistent headache, dizziness, blurred vision, lassitude, lusterless complexion, pain relieved by warmth and aggravated by cold, physical strain, or mental stress
Pulse:	Weak, thready
Tongue:	Pale body with thin, white coating
Treatment:	Supplement source qi: **CV-6**† Raise yang: **GV-20**† Reinforce kidney essence: **BL-23**† Supplement blood: **BL-18, BL-20, ST-36**

Facial Pain

Invasion of Wind-Cold Pathogen

Symptoms:	Abrupt onset, "electric shock" pain sensation, or boring, stabbing, intolerable pain that is transient and paroxysmal. Often accompanied by local spasm, running nose and tearing, salivation
Pulse:	Wiry, tight
Tongue:	Pale body, thin, white coat
Treatment:	Dispel wind pathogen: **TB-5, GB-20,** and add points according to area affected below

Hepatogastric Fire Effulgence

Symptoms:	Pain accompanied by irritability, thirst, constipation
Pulse:	Wiry, rapid
Tongue:	Dry, yellow coating
Treatment:	Calm liver and stomach fire: **LV-2, LV-3, ST-44,** and add points according to area affected below

Yin Depletion Fire Effulgence

Symptoms:	Pain of insidious onset, emaciation, malar flush, lumbar soreness, lassitude, aggravated by fatigue
Pulse:	Thready, rapid
Tongue:	Red body with little or no coating
Treatment:	Supplement yin to reduce fire: **KI-6, SP-6** Add points according to area affected

Trigeminal Neuralgia

Symptoms:	Transient, paroxysmal pain on facial regions supplied by different branches of trigeminal nerve. Treat points according to the branch affected
Treatment:	1st (ophthalmic) branch: **TB-5, GB-14, H-HN-9** (*taiyang*)**, BL-2** 2nd (maxillary) branch: **LI-4, ST-2, ST-3, GV-26** 3rd (mandibular) branch: **ST-44, ST-7, ST-6, CV-24**

Syncope

Depletion

Symptoms:	Shallow breathing, mouth agape, perspiration, pallor, cold extremities
Pulse:	Deep, feeble, thready
Treatment:	General resuscitation: **GV-26, PC-9** Recapture qi, reestablish yang: **GV-20, CV-6, ST-36**

CAM substitutes **PC-6** for **PC-9**. This is clinically unsound and may be a misprint

Repletion

Symptoms:	Coarse breathing, rigid extremities, clenched jaws
Pulse:	Deep, wiry *Tongue:* Red or somber purple
Treatment:	General resuscitation: **GV-26, PC-9** Dissipate heat, clear mind: **PC-8, KI-1** Normalize circulation of qi and blood by clearing the channels: **LI-4, LV-3**

Dizziness and Vertigo

Symptoms:	Giddiness, blurring of vision, whirling sensation, tendency to fall

Ascendant Hyperactivity of Liver Yang

Symptoms:	Dizziness aggravated by anger, irritability, tinnitus, flushed face, red eyes, nausea, backache, bitter taste in mouth, dream-disturbed sleep.
Pulse:	Wiry, rapid *Tongue:* Red body with yellow coating
Treatment:	Strengthen kidney: **BL-23, KI-3** Calm liver yang: **LV-2, BL-18, GB-20**

Interior Retention of Phlegm-Damp

Symptoms:	Pallor, lusterless complexion, weakness, listlessness, lassitude, palpitation, insomnia, pale lips and nails
Pulse:	Thready, weak *Tongue:* Pale body
Treatment:	Strengthen vital energy: **CV-4**† Raise yang qi: **GV-20**† Invigorate spleen and stomach: **BL-20**†, **ST-36**†, **SP-6**†

19   Selected Miscellaneous Disorders

Appendicitis	
General Symptoms:	Abdominal pain with tenderness, aggravated by coughing or flexing right leg. Eventually localizes in lower right abdominal quadrant, with particular pain at McBurney's point. May be accompanied by constipation.
Pulse:	Forceful, rapid
Tongue:	Thick, sticky yellow coating
Treatment:	Empirical point for appendicitis: **M-LE-13** (*lanwei*) Cool intestinal heat: **LI-11** Clear stagnation in large intestine: **ST-25, ST-37** Reduce fever: **LI-4, GV-14** Calm stomach and check vomiting: **PC-6, CV-12**

Goiter	
General Symptoms:	Swelling of neck; possibly accompanied by oppression in chest, palpitation, dyspnea, hoarse voice, exophthalmos, irritability, anxiety, sweating
Pulse:	Wiry, slippery, rapid
Treatment:	Clear and discharge stagnant qi and phlegm: **TB-13** Promote circulation of qi and blood in local area: **LI-17, SI-17, CV-22** Promote circulation of qi and blood in yangming channels: **LI-4, ST-36**
Supplementary treatment by symptom:	Liver qi stagnation: **LV-3, CV-17** Palpitations: **PC-6, HT-7** Exophthalmos: **TB-23, BL-2, BL-1, GB-20** Irritability, anxiety, and sweating: **SP-6, KI-7**

Sunstroke	
General Symptoms:	Headache, hidrosis, thirst, collapse, sudden loss of consciousness
Mild Type	
Pulse:	Floating, large, rapid
Treatment:	Drain heat: **GV·14, PC-7, BL-40** (bleed) Reduce fever: **LI-4, LI-11**
Severe Type	
Pulse:	Deep, forceless
Treatment:	Resuscitate and clear the mind: **GV-26, GV-20** Reduce heat: **PC-3, BL-40** (bleed), **M-UE-1-5** (*shixuan*) (bleed)

Malaria	
Symptoms:	Intermittent waves of chills and fever, with headache, flushed face, thirst; may be accompanied by stifling oppression in chest and hypochondrium, bitter taste in mouth
Pulse:	Wiry, rapid *Tongue:* Yellow, sticky, thin coat
Treatment:	Remove obstruction and heat in governing vessel: **GV-14, GV-13** Harmonize qi in shaoyang channels: **TB-2, GB-41** Activate circulation in taiyang and governing vessel to expel pathogen: **SI-3** Eliminate interior heat: **PC-5**
Supplementary treatment according to symptom:	High fever: **LI-11** Mass in right hypochondrium: **LV-13, BL-51†, M-BW-16†** *(pigen)* Severe attack with delirium: bleed 12 jing-well points of the hands

Halitosis	
Symptoms:	Foul-smelling breath
Pulse:	Rapid *Tongue:* Yellow fur
Treatment:	Clear and discharge stagnant qi and phlegm: **TB-13** Promote circulation of qi and blood in local area: **LI-17, SI-17, CV-22** Promote circulation of qi and blood in yangming channels: **LI-4, ST-36**

Insomnia

General Treatment:	Calm the spirit: **HT-7** Support blood: **PC-6** Regulate yin: **SP-6**

Spleen and Blood Insufficiency

Symptoms:	Difficulty in falling asleep, disturbed sleep; accompanied by palpitation, poor memory, lassitude, listlessness, anorexia, sallow complexion
Pulse:	Thready, weak *Tongue:* Pale body with thin coating
Treatment:	Support blood management and production: **BL-20, BL-15** Calm dream-disturbed sleep: **SP-1**†

Breakdown of Cardiorenal Interaction

Symptoms:	Irritability and insomnia, accompanied by dizziness, tinnitus, low back pain, dry mouth, palpitation, "fever in five hearts" (burning sensation in chest, palms, and soles), nocturnal emission, poor memory
Pulse:	Thready, rapid *Tongue:* Red body
Treatment:	Adjust the heart and kidney disharmony: **BL-15, BL-23, KI-3**

Upflaming of Liver Fire

Symptoms:	Mental depression, irritability, dream-disturbed sleep; accompanied by headache, distending pain in costal and hypochondriac region, bitter taste in mouth
Pulse:	Wiry *Tongue:* Red body
Treatment:	Calm liver and gallbladder: **BL-18, BL-19** Clear liver fire in head: **GB-12**

Stomach Dysfunction

Symptoms:	Insomnia accompanied by epigastric fullness and discomfort, abdominal distention, eructation, difficult defecation
Pulse:	Full, forceful, rolling *Tongue:* Sticky coating
Treatment:	Harmonize digestion: **BL-21, ST-36**

Hiccough	
General Treatment:	Relieve epigastric fullness: **PC-6** Promote descending function of stomach: **CV-12, ST-36** Subdue ascending qi: **BL-17, CV-22**

Food Retention

Symptoms:	Loud hiccough, epigastric and abdominal distention, anorexia
Pulse:	Rolling, forceful
Tongue:	Thick, sticky coating
Treatment:	Ease chest and diaphragm: **CV-14** Relieve abdominal stagnation: **ST-44**

Qi Stagnation

Symptoms:	Continual hiccough, distention and oppression in chest and hypochondrium
Pulse:	Wiry, forceful
Tongue:	Thin coating
Treatment:	Disperse stagnant qi in upper burner: **CV-17** Calm liver to relax diaphragm: **LV-3, LV-14**

Pathogenic Cold in Stomach

Symptoms:	Slow, forceful hiccough, possibly alleviated by hot drinks, aggravated by cold, epigastric discomfort
Pulse:	Slow
Tongue:	White, moist coating
Treatment:	Warm spleen and stomach to eliminate cold: **CV-13†**

Edema
Repletion (Yang Edema)
Symptoms: Abrupt onset; first appears on head, face, or lower extremities; lustrous skin. Possibly accompanied by cough, asthma, fever, thirst, scant urine, or low back pain.
Pulse: Floating, or rolling and rapid
Tongue: Thin, white coating
Treatment: *Edema above the waist:* Promote perspiration by activating lung qi: **LU-7, LI-4**   *Edema below the waist:* Promote diuresis to eliminate damp: **LI-6, SP-9, BL-28**
Depletion (Yin edema)
Symptoms: Insidious onset; first appears on pedis dorsum or eyelids, then over entire body. May be accompanied by chilliness, pallor, backache, general weakness, abdominal distention, loose stools
Pulse: Deep, thready
Tongue: Pale body with white coating
Treatment: Supplement spleen and kidney yang: **BL-20†, BL-23†**   Supplement qi and move water: **CV-6†, CV-9†**   Remove obstruction from water passages: **BL-39**   Reinforce stomach and spleen to transform damp: **ST-36†, SP-6**
Treatment according to symptom: Edema of the face: **GV-26**   Constipation with abdominal distention: **ST-40**   Edema of the pedis dorsum: **GB-41, SP-5**

Gallstones	
General Symptoms:	Sudden, intense cramping pain in the right hypochondrium, possibly radiating to the right shoulder. May be accompanied by chills, vomiting, persipiration, and loss of consciousness.
Pulse:	Deep, tight, bound
Tongue:	Yellow fur
Treatment:	Accelerate passage of stones: **LV-14, BL-18, GB-24, BL-19** (all points right side only; electrical stimulation is recommended) Prevent formation of new stones: **BL-22, LI-11, PC-4, ST-36, GB-34**

Kidney Stones	
Symptoms:	Dull or twisting pain in the area of the kidneys, at times radiating to the abdomen and reproductive organs; when extreme, cramping pain radiating to the medial thigh. May be accompanied by nausea and vomiting. During periods of no pain, the kidneys may be painful when palpated.
Treatment:	Dissolve and clear stones: **BL-23†, BL-28†, GB-34†, GV-4†** (daily treatment)

Body Odor	
Symptoms:	Ammonia-like stench, particularly from the armpits; more pronounced in summer
Treatment:	Regulate perspiration in armpits: even movement (neither supplementing nor draining) needling at **GB-21**, then drain **ST-36**

120

Jaundice	
General Treatment:	Fortify spleen to dispel damp: **SP-9, ST-36** Supplement gallbladder: **GB-24, BL-19, BL-48, GV-9**
Yang (Damp-Heat) Jaundice	
Symptoms:	Bright yellow skin, yellow sclerae, dark urine, fever, heavy sensation of the body, thirst, abdominal fullness
Pulse:	Wiry, rapid *Tongue:* Yellow, sticky coating
Treatment:	Dispel hepatocystic damp-heat: **LV-3** (direct needle toward **KI-1**), **GB-34**
Yin (Cold-Damp) Jaundice	
Symptoms:	Lusterless yellow skin, yellow sclerae, dark urine, with heavy sensation in body, lassitude, somnolence, absence of thirst
Pulse:	Deep, slow *Tongue:* Thick, white coating
Treatment:	Fortify spleen to dispel cold and damp: **BL-20†, BL-48†, LV-13†**

20 Selected Emergency Treatments

<table>
<tr><td colspan="2" align="center">**Emergency Treatments**
(From *Zhenjiu Jingwei*, 429-436)</td></tr>
<tr><td align="center">**Condition**</td><td align="center">**Procedure**</td></tr>
<tr>
<td>*Shock*</td>
<td>With chills in extremities or loss of consciousness: **GV-26** (finger pressure or needle) **GV-20** (moxa); **KI-1** (needle)</td>
</tr>
<tr>
<td>*Heart Conditions*</td>
<td>Major point: **ST-36**
With palpitations or tachycardia: **PC-6, HT-7**
With difficult breathing: **LI-4**
Prophylaxis: **PC-6, PC-5, ST-36**</td>
</tr>
<tr>
<td>*Cerebral Hemorrhage (windstrike)*</td>
<td>*Tense (replete) type:* Bleed twelve jing-well points or **M-UE-1-5** (*shixuan*), then drain **LI-4, ST-36, LV-3**

Flaccid (deplete) type: Supplement **GV-26, GV-20** (moxa), **KI-1** (moxa), then supplement **LI-4, PC-6, ST-36**</td>
</tr>
<tr>
<td>*Serious Bleeding*</td>
<td>Cleft-*xi* point of channel(s) involved, **SP-6**, direct moxas at **SP-1** and **LV-1**</td>
</tr>
<tr>
<td>*Hemorrhage, post-partum*</td>
<td>Direct moxas at **SP-1** and **LV-1**, then at **GV-20**</td>
</tr>
<tr>
<td>*Asthmatic crises*</td>
<td>**CV-22, CV-17, PC-5, ST-40**</td>
</tr>
<tr>
<td>*Appendicitis, acute*</td>
<td>Strong stimulation at **ST-36, M-LE-13** (*lanwei*)
Auxiliary points: nausea, **PC-6** diarrhea, **ST-25**; fever, **LI-4, LI-11**</td>
</tr>
<tr>
<td>*Cholecystitis, acute*</td>
<td>Drain **GB-34, GB-38, GB-40**, then supplement **SP-6**; or let blood from vein between **ST-40** and **GB-34** on right side</td>
</tr>
<tr>
<td>*Gastroenteritis, acute*</td>
<td>Major points: **CV-12, ST-36**
Auxiliary points: **ST-25, CV-4** (cup after needling)</td>
</tr>
<tr>
<td>*Food poisoning, bacterial*</td>
<td>Strong stimulation at **CV-12, ST-36, ST-25**;
If serious vomiting: **PC-6**;
Anal sphincter spasm: **BL-57**; lowered blood pressure: **CV-8** (salt moxa);
Auxiliary points: **BL-40** (bleed), **LU-5**</td>
</tr>
</table>

Emergency Treatments	
(Continued)	
Condition	**Procedure**
Dysentery, bacillary	Major points: **CV-12** with **ST-36**, *or* **LI-11** and **ST-37**. If high fever: **LI-4**; Nausea and vomiting: **PC-6**; Persistent urge to defecate: **ST-25, LV-3**
Rubeola (measles)	For itching and pain: **BL-67, ST-15**; then drain **BL-13, BL-60** and supplement **BL-40**. If major outbreak occurs in head and neck, add **GB-20**; for trunk or lower limbs, add **GB-31**
Headaches, severe	Unilateral: **GB-43, GB-31** Frontal: **SP-4** Temporal: **ST-43, PC-6** Occipital or vertex: **BL-65** If vision is affected add **SI-3**
Drunkenness	Rapid, strong stimulation at **GV-25**, followed by letting blood at this point.
Insomnia	Major points: **HT-7, SP-6, LI-4** If chronic: **M-HN-3** (*yintang*), **HT-7, LV-2**. Treat in evening, just before retiring, if possible.

Appendix

Selected
Point
Locations

Selected Point Locations	
Lung Channel Points	
LU-1	In the first intercostal space below the acromial extremity of the clavicle, 1 *cun* below LU-2, 6 *cun* lateral to the conception vessel.
LU-2	In the depression immediately below the acromial extremity of the clavicle, 6 *cun* lateral to the conception vessel.
LU-4	On the upper arm, 1 *cun* below LU-3, on the radial side of the biceps muscle of the arm (m. biceps brachii).
LU-5	At the cubital crease, on the radial side of the tendon of the biceps muscle of the arm (m. biceps brachii). The point is best located with the elbow slightly flexed.
LU-7	Proximal to the styloid process of the radius, 1.5 *cun* above the transverse crease of the wrist. When the thumb and index finger of each hand are interlocked, with the index finger of one hand resting on the styloid process of the other, the point is in the depression just under the tip of the index finger.
LU-9	At the transverse crease of the wrist, in the depression of the radial side of the radial artery.
LU-10	On the thenar prominence at the midpoint of the first metacarpal bone, on the border of the red and white skin.
LU-11	On the radial side of the thumb, about 0.1 *cun* proximal to the corner of the nail.
Large Intestine Channel Points	
LI-1	On the radial side of the index finger, about 0.1 *cun* proximal to the corner of the nail.
LI-2	On the radial side of the index finger, distal to the metacarpophalangeal joint, at the border of the red and white skin. The point is located with the finger slightly flexed.
LI-4	In the center of the flesh between the 1st and 2nd metacarpal bones, slightly closer to the 2nd metacarpal bone. If the transverse crease of the interphalangeal joint of the thumb of one hand is lined up with the margin of the web between the thumb and the index finger of the other hand, the point is where the tip of the thumb touches.

Large Intestine Channel Points (Continued)	
LI-10	2 *cun* below LI-11 on the line drawn from LI-5.
LI-11	When the elbow is flexed the point is in the depression at the lateral end of the transverse cubital crease, midway between LU-5 and the lateral epicondyle of the humerus.
Stomach Channel Points	
ST-4	Lateral to the corner of the mouth, directly below ST-3.
ST-6	One finger breadth anterior and superior to the lower angle of the mandible where the masseter muscle attaches. At the prominence of the muscle when the teeth are clenched.
ST-24	1 *cun* above the umbilicus, 2 *cun* lateral to CV-9.
ST-25	2 *cun* lateral to the center of the umbilicus.
ST-29	4 *cun* below the umbilicus, 2 *cun* lateral to CV-3.
ST-36	3 *cun* below ST-35, roughly 1 *cun* lateral to the crest of the tibia. If the palm of the hand is placed over the patella, the point is located at the level where the middle finger ends.
ST-37	6 *cun* below ST-35, a finger's breadth lateral to the anterior crest of the tibia.
ST-39	One finger's breadth lateral to the anterior crest of the tibia, 3 *cun* below ST-37.
ST-40	8 *cun* superior and anterior to the external malleolus, about one finger's breadth lateral to ST-38.
ST-41	At the junction of the dorsum of the foot and the leg, between the tendons of the long extensor muscle of the toes and the long extensor muscle of the great toe (m. extensor digitorum longus and m. extensor hallucis longus), approximately at the level of the tip of the external malleolus.
ST-42	At the highest point of the dorsum of the foot, in the depression between the 2nd and 3rd metatarsal bones and the cuneiform bone.
ST-44	Proximal to the web margin between the 2nd and 3rd toes, in the depression distal and lateral to the 2nd metatarsophalangeal joint.
ST-45	On the lateral side of the 2nd toe, about 0.1 *cun* proximal to the corner of the nail.

Spleen Channel Points	
SP-1	On the medial side of the big toe, about 0.1 *cun* proximal to the corner of the nail.
SP-2	On the medial side of the big toe, distal and inferior to the 1st metatarsophalangeal joint, at the border of the red and white skin.
SP-3	Proximal and inferior to the head of the 1st metatarsal bone, at the border of the red and white skin.
SP-4	In the depression distal and inferior to the base of the 1st metatarsal bone, at the border of the red and white flesh.
SP-6	3 *cun* directly above the tip of the medial malleolus, on the posterior border of the tibia, on a line drawn from the medial malleolus to SP-9.
SP-8	3 *cun* below the medial condyle of the tibia, on the line connecting SP-9 and the medial malleolus.
SP-9	On the lower border of the medial condyle of the tibia, in the depression between the posterior border of the tibia and the gastrocnemius muscle (m. gastrocnemius).
SP-10	When the knee is flexed, the point is 2 *cun* above the mediosuperior border of the patella, on the bulge of the medial portion of the quadriceps muscle of the thigh (m. vastus medialis). Another way to locate this point is to cup your right palm over the patient's left knee, with the thumb on its medial side and the four other fingers directed proximally. The point will be found where the tip of your thumb rests.
SP-11	6 *cun* above SP-10, on the line drawn from SP-10 to SP-12.
SP-13	0.7 *cun* above SP-12, 4 *cun* lateral to the midline.
Heart Channel Points	
HT-3	When the elbow is flexed, the point is at the medial end of the transverse cubital crease, in the depression anterior to the medial epicondyle of the humerus.
HT-5	1 *cun* proximal to the transverse wrist crease. On the radial side of the tendon of the ulnar flexor muscle of the wrist (m. flexor carpi ulnaris).
HT-7	On the transverse crease on the palmar side of the wrist, in the articular region between the pisiform bone and the ulna, in the depression on the radial side of the tendon of the ulnar flexor muscle of the wrist (m. flexor carpi ulnaris).

| *Heart Channel Points (Continued)*	
HT-8	On the palmar surface, between the 4th and 5th metacarpal bones. When a fist is made, the point will be found where the tip of the little finger rests.
HT-9	On the radial side of the little finger, about 0.1 *cun* proximal to the corner of the nail.
Small Intestine Channel Points	
SI-2	When a loose fist is made, the point is distal to the metacarpophalangeal joint, at the border of the red and white skin.
SI-4	On the ulnar side of the palm, in the depression between the base of the 5th metacarpal bone and the triquetral bone.
Bladder Channel Points	
BL-12	1.5 *cun* lateral to the lower border of the spinous process of the 2nd thoracic vertebra.
BL-13	1.5 *cun* lateral to the lower border of the spinous process of the 3rd thoracic vertebra.
BL-14	1.5 *cun* lateral to the lower border of the spinous process of the 4th thoracic vertebra.
BL-15	1.5 *cun* lateral to the lower border of the spinous process of the 5th thoracic vertebra.
BL-18	1.5 *cun* lateral to the lower border of the spinous process of the 9th thoracic vertebra.
BL-19	1.5 *cun* lateral to the lower border of the spinous process of the 10th thoracic vertebra.
BL-20	1.5 *cun* lateral to the lower border of the spinous process of the 11th thoracic vertebra.
BL-21	1.5 *cun* lateral to the lower border of the spinous process of the 12th thoracic vertebra.
BL-22	1.5 *cun* lateral to the lower border of the spinous process of the 1st lumbar vertebra.

Bladder Channel Points (Continued)	
BL-23	1.5 *cun* lateral to the lower border of the spinous process of the 2nd lumbar vertebra.
BL-25	1.5 *cun* lateral to the lower border of the spinous process of the 4th lumbar vertebra, approximately at the level of the upper border of the iliac crest.
BL-27	At the level of the 1st sacral foramen, 1.5 *cun* lateral to the governing vessel.
BL-28	At the level of the 2nd sacral foramen, 1.5 *cun* lateral to the governing vessel, in the depression between the medial border of the posterior superior iliac spine and the sacrum.
BL-40	At the midpoint of the transverse crease of the popliteal fossa, between the tendons of biceps muscle of the thigh (m. biceps femoris) and semitendinosus muscle (m. semitendinosus). This point is located with the patient in a prone posture or with flexed knee.
BL-58	7 *cun* above BL-60, on the posterior border of the fibula, on the lateral anterior border of the gastrocnemius muscle, about 1 *cun* inferior and lateral to BL-57.
BL-66	In the depression distal and slightly inferior to the 5th metatarsophalangeal joint.
Kidney Channel Points	
KI-1	In the depression appearing on the sole when the foot is in plantar flexion, one third of the distance from the base of the toes to the heel.
KI-3	In the depression between the medial malleolus and the Achilles tendon (t. calcaneus), level with the tip of the medial malleolus.
KI-6	1 *cun* below the medial malleolus.
KI-7	2 *cun* above KI-3, on the anterior border of the Achilles tendon (t. calcaneus).
KI-10	On the medial side of the popliteal fossa, level with BL-40, between the tendons of the semitendinosus muscle (m. semitendinosus) and the semimembranosus muscle (m. semimembranosus) when the knee is flexed.

	Pericardium Channel Points (Continued)
PC-3	At the transverse cubital crease, on the ulnar side of the tendon of biceps muscle of the arm (m. biceps brachii).
PC-5	3 *cun* above the transverse crease of the wrist, between the tendons of the long palmar muscle and the radial flexor muscle of the wrist (m. palmaris longus and m. flexor carpi radialis).
PC-6	2 *cun* above the transverse crease of the wrist, between the tendons of the long palmar muscle and the radial flexor muscle of the wrist (m. palmaris longus and m. flexor carpi radialis).
PC-7	In the depression in the middle of the transverse crease of the wrist, between the tendons of the long palmar muscle and the radial flexor muscle of the wrist (m. palmaris longus and m. flexor carpi radialis).
PC-8	On the palm of the hand between the 2nd and 3rd metacarpal bones, proximal to the metacarpophalangeal joint, on the radial side of the 3rd metacarpal bone.
PC-9	0.1 *cun* proximal to the corner of the nail on the radial side of the middle finger.
	Triple Burner Channel Points
TB-2	Proximal to the margin of the web between the ring and small fingers. The point is located with clenched fist.
TB-3	When the hand is placed with the palm facing downward, the point is on the dorsum of the hand between the 4th and 5th metacarpal bones, in the depression proximal to the metacarpophalangeal joint.
TB-5	2 *cun* above TB-4, between the radius and ulna.
TB-6	3 *cun* above TB-4, between the ulna and radius.

	Gallbladder Channel Points
GB-20	On the posterior aspect of the neck, below the occipital bone, in the depression between the sternocleidomastoid muscle (m. sterno-cleidomastoideus) and trapezius muscle (m. trapezius).
GB-24	Inferior to the nipple, between the cartilage of the 7th and 8th ribs, one rib space below and slightly lateral to LV-14.
GB-25	At the inferior border of the free end of the 12th rib.
GB-34	In the depression anterior and inferior to the head of the fibula.
GB-43	Between the 4th and 5th toes, proximal to the margin of the web.
	Liver Channel Points
LV-1	On the lateral side of the dorsum of the terminal phalanx of the great toe, between the lateral corner of the nail and interphalangeal joint.
LV-2	Between the first and second toe, proximal to the margin of the web.
LV-3	In the depression distal to the junction of the 1st and 2nd metatarsal bones.
LV-8	On the medial side of the knee joint. When the knee is bent, the point is posterior to the medial condyle of the tibia and superior to the border of the tendons of those muscles attaching at the medial side of the knee.
LV-13	Below the free end of the eleventh floating rib.
LV-14	On the mammillary line, two ribs below the nipple, in the sixth inter-costal space.

	Conception Vessel Points
CV-3	On the anterior midline, 4 *cun* below the umbilicus, 1 *cun* above the upper border of the pubic symphysis.
CV-4	On the anterior midline of the abdomen, 3 *cun* below the umbilicus.
CV-6	On the anterior midline, 1.5 *cun* below the umbilicus.
CV-8	In the center of the umbilicus.
CV-9	On the anterior midline, 1 *cun* above the umbilicus.
CV-10	On the anterior midline, 2 *cun* above the umbilicus.
CV-12	On the anterior midline, 4 *cun* above the umbilicus.
CV-13	On the anterior midline, 5 *cun* above the umbilicus.
CV-14	On the anterior midline, 6 *cun* above the umbilicus.
CV-17	On the anterior midline, between the nipples, level with the fourth intercostal space.
CV-22	On the anterior midline in the center of the suprasternal notch.
	Governing Vessel Channel Points
GV-4	Below the spinous process of the second lumbar vertebra.
GV-14	Between the spinous processes of the seventh cervical vertebra and the first thoracic vertebra, approximately at the level of the shoulder.
GV-15	On the posterior midline, 0.5 *cun* below GV-16 in the depression 0.5 *cun* within the hairline.
GV-16	Directly below the external occipital protuberance, in the depression between the attachments of the trapezius muscle (m. trapezius).
GV-26	Below the nose, a little above the midpoint of the philtrum.

Non-Channel Points	
M-HN-3	At the midpoint between the eyebrows *(yintanga)*.
M-HN-20a+b	On the veins on either side of the vinculum linguae: *jinjin* (left), and yuye (right).
M-HN-6	In the hollow in the middle of the eyebrow, directly above the pupil when the eyes gaze straight ahead *(yuyao)*.
M-HN-8	Approximately one quarter the distance from the lateral to the medial side of the orbit, at the inferior border *(qiuhou)*.
M-HN-9	On the temple, approximately one *cun* posterior to the midpoint between the outer canthus and the tip of the eyebrow *(taiyang)*.
M-CA-18	Four *cun* below the navel, three *cun* lateral to CV-3 *(zigong)*.
M-BW-1b	Approximately one *cun* lateral to the spinous process of the 7th cervical vertebra *(dingchuan)*.
M-BW-16	Three and a half *cun* lateral to the spinous process of the 1st lumbar vertebra *(pigen)*.
M-BW-24	In the depression 4 *cun* lateral to the lower end of the spinous process of the 3rd lumbar vertebra *(yaoyan)*.
M-BW-25	In the depression below the spinous process of the 5th lumbar vertebra *(shiqizhuxia)*.
M-BW-35	48 individual points located on both sides of each vertebra, ½ to 1 cun lateral to the midline of the spine *(jiaji)*.
M-UE-1	Ten individual points, each on the middle of the tip of each finger, about 0.1 *cun* from the fingernail *(shixuan)*.
M-UE-9	Eight points, each on the palmer surface of the four fingers (not the thumb), at the midpoint of the transverse crease of each proximal phalangeal joint *(sifeng)*.
M-UE-19	Three points, located on the dorsum of the hand at the articulations of the 2nd and 3rd, 3rd and 4th, and 4th and 5th metacarpal bones *(yaotong)*.

	Non-Channel Points (Continued)
M-UE-22	Eight individual points, each located in the depression immediately behind and between the metacarpophalangeal joints on the back of each hand *(shangbaxia)*.
M-UE-24	On the dorsum of the hand, approximately 0.5 *cun* proximal to and between the metacarpophalangeal joints of the 2nd and 3rd metacarpal bones *(luozhen)*.
M-LE-8	Eight points, each in the web between each toe *(bafeng)*.
M-LE-13	Approximately 2 *cun* below ST-36 *(lanweixue)*.
M-LE-16	Lateral "eye-of-knee": when the knee is flexed, in the large hollow below the kneecap on the lateral side of the patellar tendon *(dubai)*.
M-LE-27	In the depression at the middle of the superior margin of the patella *(heding)*.
M-LE-34	One *cun* above SP-10 *(baichongwo)*.

Bibliography

Beijing Institute of Traditional Chinese Medicine, et al. *Zhongguo Zhenjiuxue Gaiyao* (Essentials of Chinese Acupuncture). Beijing: People's Health Press, 1980.

Chen-chiu Ta-ch'eng Chiao-shih (Corrected and Explained 'Great Compendium of Acumoxa'). No editors listed. Taipei: Ch'i-yeh Publishing, 1987.

Cheng Weifen, et al. *Cheng Dan'an Zhenjiu Xuanji* (Selections from Cheng Dan'an's Acupuncture). Shanghai: Science and Technology Press, 1986.

Chuang Yu-min. *Chung-kuo Chen-chiu Hsueh Chi-pen Chiao-ts'ai* (Fundamental Teaching Material of Chinese Acupuncture). Taichung: Chung-kuo I-yao Hsueh-yuen Tung-shih-hui, 1977.

Chung-i Cheng-chuang Chien-pieh Chen-tuan Hsueh (Differential Diagnosis in Chinese Medicine). No editors listed. Taipei: Ch'i-yeh Publishing, 1985.

Deng Liangyue, et al. *Zhongguo Zhenjiuxue* (Chinese Acupuncture and Moxibustion). Cheng Xinnong, ed. Beijing: Foreign Languages Press, 1987.

Huang Wei-san. *Chen-chiu K'o-hsueh* (Acupuncture Science). Taipei: Published by the author, 1972.

Liu Fei-pai. *Chung-i Nei-k'o Hsueh* (Chinese Internal Medicine). Taipei: Wu-chou Publishing, 1984.

Nanjing Institute of Traditional Chinese Medicine. *Zhongyixue Gailun* (Introduction to Chinese Medicine). Beijing: People's Health Press, 1959.

Shanghai Institute of Traditional Chinese Medicine. *Zhongyixue Jichu* (Fundamentals of Chinese Medicine). Beijing: People's Health Press, 1975.

Index